Clinical Laboratory Methods

a LANGE medical book

Clinical Laboratory Methods

Atlas of Commonly Performed Tests

Written by
Michael Laposata
Peter McCaffrey

New York   Chicago   San Francisco   Athens   Lisbon   Madrid
Mexico City   Milan   New Delhi   Singapore   Sydney   Toronto

1 2 3 4 5 6 7 8 9   DSS   26 25 24 23 22 21

ISBN 978-1-260-47028-4
MHID 1-260-47028-8

This book was set in Minion by MPS Limited.
The editors were Michael Weitz and Peter J. Boyle.
The production supervisor was Richard Ruzycka.
Project management was provided by Adwiti Pradhan and Anamika Singh, MPS Limited.

Cataloging-in-publication data for this book is on file at the Library of Congress.

McGraw Hill books are available at special quantity discounts to use as premiums and sales promotions or for use in corporate training programs. To contact a representative, please visit the Contact Us pages at www.mhprofessional.com.

To my grandparents whose bravery more than 100 years ago to immigrate to the United States has provided our entire family with opportunities that those who made the voyage could never have imagined.

ML

To my children, Briar, Huxley, and Hollis, whose books I one day hope to read.

PM

Contents

Preface

When the Robbins *Pathologic Basis of Disease* book emerged from its early editions and became increasingly larger, there was a call to make a shorter version of the textbook. What resulted was an additional book affectionately known as "Mini-Robbins" by many. It was well received by students, one of whom was me. This experiment has in retrospect indicated to me that books derived from a larger, more comprehensive book may be worth producing. *Laposata's Laboratory Medicine* has several obviously useful derivative products. McGraw Hill first produced a series of flashcards about the selection and interpretation of clinical laboratory tests. This current book focused on testing methods in the clinical laboratory is another product, with special value for medical students and practitioners of clinical laboratory science (a.k.a., medical technology). As we have learned in 2020, the choice of the method to detect SARS-CoV2 has a major impact on whether the result is a true-negative or a false-negative. This important methodologic information about each individual test was not well understood by healthcare providers at large, and had it been, it is likely to have benefited the millions who became sick and the hundreds of thousands who have perished.

This book on laboratory methods provides an overview of laboratory testing, followed by descriptions and easy-to-understand graphics for more than 60 commonly used methods. The 3rd edition of *Laposata's Laboratory Medicine* does not include the depth and breadth of chromosomal and molecular genetic methods that are carefully described in this book.

If you are searching for a publication to teach you about the clinical laboratory assays that you will need to understand to make important clinical decisions, or maybe even perform yourself, we hope that this is the text that will help you best learn about the tests.

Michael Laposata
Peter McCaffrey
Galveston, Texas, 2021

Acknowledgments

The authors would like to acknowledge Drs. Paul Steele and James H. Nichols who provided several graphics in the second chapter of the 3rd edition of *Laposata's Laboratory Medicine* which are also included in this book.

We would also like to acknowledge the editors of this book from McGraw Hill, Michael Weitz and Peter J. Boyle, whose quick responses to our many queries was extremely valuable in maintaining our momentum.

Introduction: Concepts in Clinical Laboratory Testing

THE MOST IMPORTANT CONCEPT ABOUT DIAGNOSTIC TESTING

The method used to perform a measurement of a compound in a biological sample is extremely important to know so that it is possible to determine if the result reflects the true value in the body of the patient. Knowledge of methodologic details is also required to understand the many variables that can make the result incorrect and clinically misleading.

THE EVOLUTION OF LABORATORY TESTING FROM MANUAL TO AUTOMATED METHODS

Laboratory testing was performed for decades with no instrumentation in the laboratory. All of the tests were individually developed, often locally by the laboratory director, and performed manually. Prior to the 1970s, it was not uncommon to create a standard curve for glucose measurement by pipetting increasing amounts of glucose into a series of tubes with reagents, plotting the optical density to create a standard curve on graph paper, and then measuring the amount of glucose in the sample by obtaining the optical density of the patient specimen and using the standard curve. Automation of test performance began in the 1960s and 1970s, and then has continued to increase. Tests which are not fully automated are often partially automated. The methods which are fully manual at this point are far fewer than those which are fully or partially automated. The methods described in this text are largely automated to at least some degree. The details of instrument performance and the chemistry of the reactions are depicted in the figures. The methodology, the reagents used, and the instrument all have an impact on the outcome of the test. It is for this reason that healthcare providers and especially experts in laboratory medicine must be fully aware of the methodology implemented for testing and the impact of the methodology on the test result.

THE DRAMATIC CHANGE IN THE ROLE OF THE CLINICAL LABORATORY SCIENTIST

When manual methods dominated in most clinical laboratories, the clinical laboratory scientist was almost completely focused on the analytical performance of the test. When automated instruments arrived in the laboratory, the laboratory scientist at the bench had to develop new skills that focused on demonstrating that the instrument was generating accurate test results. The need for a high level of technical competence became required because so much of the testing in the clinical laboratory was being performed on increasingly sophisticated instruments. At this time, the clinical laboratory scientist not only has to assure functional performance of testing instruments, but because there are so many tests which are highly complex, consultation by clinical laboratory scientists with patient facing healthcare providers on test selection and result interpretation is increasingly necessary. If a sample for glucose measurement was collected in a vacuum tube without a glycolysis inhibitor (a gray top tube), and the sample was transported over an 8-hour route before it arrived in the laboratory, the glucose is likely to be artefactually low because of the metabolism of the glucose by the platelets and the white blood cells prior to analysis. A practicing doctor is unlikely to know that the low glucose value is not reflective of hypoglycemia in the patient, but instead represents a preanalytical error. Communication between the clinical laboratory scientist and the healthcare provider, in this example to avoid a false diagnosis of hypoglycemia, is essential to establishing a correct diagnosis.

THE INCREASING USE OF GENETIC TESTING

When a genetic cause for cystic fibrosis was first described in the late 1980s, one mutation in one individual gene was associated with cystic fibrosis. Now more than 2000 different mutations have been found in that one gene, and the genetic classification of cystic fibrosis has produced six major types of the disease, which are treated with different highly expensive medications. What was once a disease thought to be diagnosable with a test for sweat chloride is now a disorder which requires complex genetic analysis. "Molecular" methods (this generally refers to molecular genetic methods, when, in fact, most assays measure the amount of "molecules") are highly complex and usually quite expensive. Now, for many diseases, it is possible to do one expensive genetic test to make a definitive diagnosis that stands for a lifetime, as opposed to performing many simpler tests that *suggest* a diagnosis, but never actually establish it. Experts in laboratory medicine who can communicate the results of genetic tests to a well-intended patient facing provider with only a modest understanding of genetic terminology produces an extraordinary benefit for the patient.

POINT-OF-CARE TESTING METHODS—SPEED AT THE COST OF SENSITIVITY, AND VARIABILITY BETWEEN INSTRUMENTS

The use of point-of-care testing for many compounds other than glucose has often been a matter of some controversy. It is challenging for individuals working in a clinical laboratory to understand that a person with poor eyesight and limited dexterity, and possibly even having difficulty understanding simple instructions, can effectively use a small plastic kit. It must be recognized that performing a test and making a mistake that can produce the wrong result can have lethal consequences. The methodologies used for point-of-care testing are by necessity simpler than the methodologies used in the clinical laboratory itself. For example, the test for the international normalized ratio (INR) for a patient monitoring the effects of the drug warfarin on a point-of-care device involves the use of very different reagents from those used within the clinical laboratory. For the point-of-care test, a capillary blood sample from a finger stick is used to determine the INR, and in the clinical laboratory, venous blood collected in a vacuum tube containing citrate as an anticoagulant is used. It is not uncommon to have a correction factor modify the result from a point-of-care instrument to make it more similar to the result generated in a clinical laboratory.

It is also a matter of controversy if a test that can be performed more often, even if it is less likely to be correct, may be of more benefit than a clinical laboratory test which requires much longer to generate a result. One example is the use of a test to detect antigens for SARS-CoV2 performed by the patient at low cost multiple times in a week. This is in comparison to a laboratory-based polymerase chain reaction (PCR) test which may require as many as 7–10 days to provide a result, though with a higher sensitivity to detect a SARS-CoV2 infection. Even if the PCR result is more accurate, some argue that it is clinically more beneficial to perform a less sensitive test every day. This is because during the week of waiting for the PCR test result, a patient infected with SARS-CoV2 may experience at least one positive test result using the less sensitive antigen test.

In general, the cost per test is much greater for reagents in point-of-care testing. A test that costs $50 in a drugstore to be performed by the patient as a point-of-care test can easily cost less than $10 in reagents for the same test performed in a clinical laboratory.

VARIABILITY IN TEST RESULTS USING THE SAME SAMPLE WHEN DIFFERENT METHODS, REAGENTS, OR INSTRUMENTS ARE USED

An excellent example of variability in the "same" test methodology is the PCR test for SARS-CoV2 RNA. There are literally dozens of available PCR tests, but they can vary substantially in methodology. This is because of differences in the primers and probes used as reagents, or in the individual steps in the test for SARS-CoV2 RNA. Some of the available PCR tests have the ability to detect as little as 600 nucleic acid units of the RNA per mL, and other assays are not able to detect SARS-CoV2 RNA unless there are at least 300,000 nucleic acid units per mL. This 5000-fold difference in sensitivity is clearly influential in deciding whether a patient is infected, especially for those who have a low-to-moderate amount of virus in the sample. One of the more insensitive tests for SARS-CoV2 RNA is genetic but has a methodological difference from classical PCR that allows it to have a rapid turnaround time and be used at the point of care. In general, optimizations for speed of test performance to shorten turnaround time increase simplicity of performance or reduce invasiveness of sample collection (sample collection from the nasopharynx is more invasive than collection of saliva). Such optimizations

have all been incorporated into methods to detect SARS-CoV2 RNA rapidly at the expense of reduced sensitivity. Very few practicing doctors are made aware of the methods performed in the laboratories which they use, and even if they are aware, the clinical implications of using a particular method are usually not made known to them.

DETERMINATION OF A REFERENCE RANGE AND A THRESHOLD VALUE

For many compounds measured in a clinical laboratory, it is possible to obtain biological samples from 20 or more individuals without disease, on no medications with no other variables that would influence the result of the compound being quantitated. Statistical assessment of the middle 95% of a Gaussian distributed range can easily be performed to establish a reference range. This within laboratory generation of a reference range removes some of the variables which might be present for a reference range established from individuals who might be different in some way. For example, dietary preferences that influence laboratory tests may be significantly different in one population versus another. In the 1980s, it was realized that the middle 95% of an Asian population demonstrated a much lower total cholesterol value than the middle 95% from a population in the United States. This was quite certainly a result of differences in intake of dietary fat.

With smaller clinical laboratories, and certainly for doctor's office laboratories and point-of-care testing, it is too difficult to create a locally validated reference range. For that reason, use of the reference range provided by the manufacturer is a common practice.

For some tests, there is a threshold value rather than a reference range. In some tests, the high value is abnormal, while in others the low value is abnormal. The threshold value itself varies by methodology. For some time, healthcare providers were aware of a certain threshold below which a D-dimer level ruled out a deep vein thrombosis or pulmonary embolism. As new methods appeared to measure D-dimer, the threshold values of the new methods were different from the one first introduced and remembered by clinicians evaluating patients who may have a thrombotic event. Because the practitioners had become used to a specific threshold value, the methods introduced shortly after the original D-dimer assays incorporated an artificial multiplication factor to create a result that would be less likely to be misinterpreted.

PROFICIENCY TESTING TO INCREASE THE LIKELIHOOD OF ANALYTICAL ACCURACY

To perform proficiency testing, a clinical laboratory purchases samples with known amounts of specific compounds through a program that supplies them to the laboratory on a regular basis. Proficiency testing is absolutely necessary to prove that the analytical phase of testing in a given laboratory is at least approximately correct. Proficiency testing does not establish a reference range. Proficiency testing establishes whether a laboratory is providing correct measurements for the samples sent to the laboratory for testing. The results of the proficiency test measurements are sent to a team which performs a complex statistical analysis of the data. The goal of the analysis is to compare test results from laboratories in which the reagents and instruments are the same. In this way, the proficiency testing process avoids making inappropriate comparisons between laboratories that use reagents or instruments which are not the same. The licensing of laboratories to perform tests and bill for the results is highly dependent upon success with proficiency testing, as it is a major portion of the laboratory inspection. Maintaining the integrity of samples in shipping and handling is a major task for those who manage and sell proficiency tests samples.

Companies that sell proficiency test samples do not sell samples for every possible measurement, often because they do not have a central group which can define what the acceptable range or threshold should be. To know with confidence that all test results generated in a clinical laboratory are correct, it is necessary to document an analysis of some kind which demonstrates accuracy for whatever is being measured.

PREANALYTICAL ERRORS MISTAKEN AS LABORATORY ERRORS TO THE PATIENT FACING HEALTHCARE PROVIDER

When a lab test result is unexpected by healthcare provider, a common interpretation is that the laboratory made some kind of error in the analysis of the specimen. In fact, that is not true for the vast majority of such cases. The assays now are so reproducible, especially the automated ones, that analytical errors are much less common than errors that occur before the sample is ever tested. These are called preanalytical errors. For example, for some tests the patients must be fasting; for other tests the samples must be collected in a specific vacuum tube with an anticoagulant; and for some tests the sample must be kept on ice during transportation. If there is a mistake in any of these steps, the error occurs before the test is ever performed, and that is why it is known as preanalytical. To the practicing doctor, the failure to instruct the patient to fast for at least 12 hours before a sample is collected, which produces a result that makes no medical sense for the patient's condition, is most often perceived as an analytical failure in the clinical laboratory. Therefore, it is important to know that selection of an optimal methodology, even with a flawless measurement, does not guarantee that a patient's measured result will represent what is actually present in the patient's body because preanalytical errors are extremely common.

SENDING LABORATORY TESTS TO COMMERCIAL LABORATORIES WITH AWARENESS OF METHODOLOGIES

Some patients will need a test that is too complex to be performed in a nearby laboratory to establish or to rule out a diagnosis. This is true for large and small laboratories because no laboratory performs every available laboratory test. Selecting a single commercial laboratory for most tests that must be sent out is a major decision which involves, among other variables, the methods used to perform measurements. It is important to know which methods are used by the commercial laboratory, so that the results are understood by the laboratory scientists at the laboratory from which the sample was sent. Issues like potential interferences that affect a particular laboratory test can then be communicated to the ordering provider. The preanalytical, analytical, and postanalytical phases are emphasized to different extents by the major commercial laboratories. The choice of a low-cost provider can have negative clinical impact if the commercial laboratory is not willing to pay attention to all the details that will affect the test result. For example, a vacuum tube filled with blood anticoagulated with citrate (a blue top tube), submitted for performance of coagulation testing, must have the tests run within a limited number of hours from the time of collection. If the commercial laboratory allows such samples to sit overnight, it will provide inaccurate results that could alter, for example, the dose of an anticoagulant, and permit a patient to suffer a bleeding or thrombotic disorder. Another critical point about tests that a clinical laboratory may perform in low volume is that for some of these, the results are needed as soon as possible for both quality of care and cost considerations. An example of this is a test for heparin-induced thrombocytopenia. If the patient has this condition, the treatment involves substitution of heparin with a very expensive alternative anticoagulant. It can cost hundreds of thousands of dollars for this alternative anticoagulant to be used while waiting for a test result from a commercial laboratory. For that reason, maintaining a test which is not often performed in a clinical laboratory for a typically urgent decision makes both clinical and financial sense.

UNDERSTANDING THE FIGURES DEPICTING EACH METHOD

The methods described in this book are predominantly the common ones found in clinical laboratories. Each method description provides an overview of the basic concept of the assay, minimizing the details, while including clinically important information and a comment on the expense of the test and the complexity of the assay in the laboratory.

Each method also has a descriptor to reflect whether it is manual, semiautomated, or highly automated. A comment has been added if microscopy is involved, as this makes any technique highly manual. It should be noted that for some methods, there is an option for manual performance or for using some level of automation. There is usually greater automation in the larger clinical laboratories because larger laboratories are more likely to have the test volume and the financial resources to justify the automated option. The purchase of test reagents in large quantities also results in a lower purchase price. The term "semiautomated" indicates that there is a manual component associated with the use of an instrument that performs some steps of the analysis.

The expense assessment attached to each assay described in this chapter is an approximation, listed as low, moderate, or high. The charge for the test set by the institution operating the laboratory is usually proportional to the expense of the reagents, supplies, and labor required to perform the test. On occasion, however, there is a great disparity between the actual expense to perform the test and the amount charged by the institution for the assay. With this in mind, the expense estimation provided for each method in this chapter is more closely related to the actual cost of reagents, supplies, and labor in the laboratory, with the understanding that the amount charged for the test should be in the same range of low, moderate, or high—but it is not always the case.

The turnaround time for an assay is not provided because it is impossible to know all of the elements associated with the turnaround time for a test within an individual institution. Broadly speaking, the turnaround time is shorter for assays that are highly automated and less expensive, and longer for assays that are manual and highly expensive. It is important to understand that the turnaround time for an assay can be calculated using different starting points. For example, one starting point is the time a sample is collected. Another starting point is the time that a sample enters the laboratory. However, the most relevant starting time clinically, which predates the previous two starting times, is the time at which the physician actually orders the test. Similarly, there are different end points in the assessment of turnaround time. Most commonly, the end point is the time at which the result is reported by the laboratory into the laboratory information system. However, it is most important to know when the physician becomes aware of the result, because it is at that point that treatment may commence.

Finally, it should be noted what methods are not presented in this chapter. There are a number of methods that have been used progressively less over time, and in many institutions these assays are no longer performed at all in the clinical laboratory. These are numerous and include, among many, the radioimmunoassay (RIA), immunoelectrophoresis, lipoprotein electrophoresis, and the bleeding time. A major effort was made to greatly expand the number of molecular genetic methods. These molecular genetic methods are described in this book. These are often highly complex, and the intention was to provide enough detail for the methods to be understood without making them confusing at the same time.

Clinical Laboratory Methods

INDIVIDUAL
METHODS
DESCRIPTIONS

1 Methods in Clinical Immunology

ANTINUCLEAR ANTIBODY (ANA) TESTING

A sample of diluted patient serum is added to a monolayer of cells on a glass slide. If there are antibodies in the patient's serum to an antigen in the nuclei of the cells on the slide, they will become bound. A fluorescent-labeled anti-IgG antibody is then added to detect antibody from the patient serum that has become bound to the cell nuclei. The specimen is reviewed by fluorescence microscopy. Information about the presence of antinuclear antibody is obtained in this test, and specific autoimmune disorders may be identified from the pattern of nuclear staining observed microscopically. Common nuclear staining patterns include rimmed (peripheral), homogeneous (diffuse), speckled, and nucleolar, along with others.

Antinuclear antibody (ANA) testing

To screen for autoimmune disorders by identifying antibodies which bind to the nucleus within cells in a specific pattern

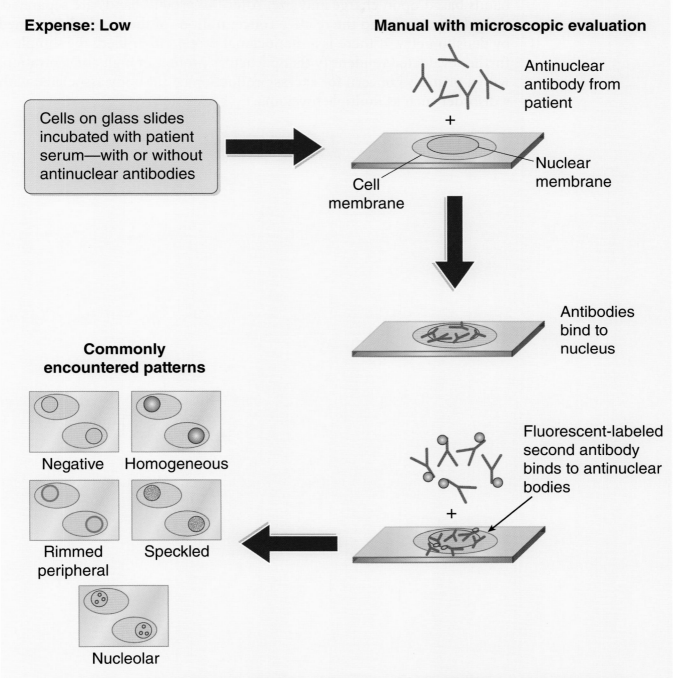

Expense: Low

Manual with microscopic evaluation

Antinuclear antibody from patient

+

Cells on glass slides incubated with patient serum—with or without antinuclear antibodies

Cell membrane

Nuclear membrane

Antibodies bind to nucleus

Commonly encountered patterns

Negative   Homogeneous

Rimmed peripheral   Speckled

Nucleolar

Fluorescent-labeled second antibody binds to antinuclear bodies

+

If an antibody is detected, the patient's serum is progressively diluted until the staining is no longer detected. The final result includes the highest serum dilution producing a detectable response and the pattern of nuclear staining.

PROTEIN ELECTROPHORESIS (PEP)

Samples containing protein subjected to electrophoresis include serum, concentrated urine, and concentrated cerebrospinal fluid. The samples are applied to a gel, and the proteins in the specimen are separated into distinct bands based upon charge and size. After the protein bands are separated, the gel is stained, and the relative concentrations of the bands determined by densitometry. If there is a monoclonal protein identified, the sample is further evaluated to identify that particular protein in high concentration, with a primary concern for excess production of antibody associated with a disorder such as multiple myeloma.

Protein electrophoresis (PEP)

To identify a monoclonal protein in blood, urine, or cerebrospinal fluid by separating it from normal proteins by electrophoresis

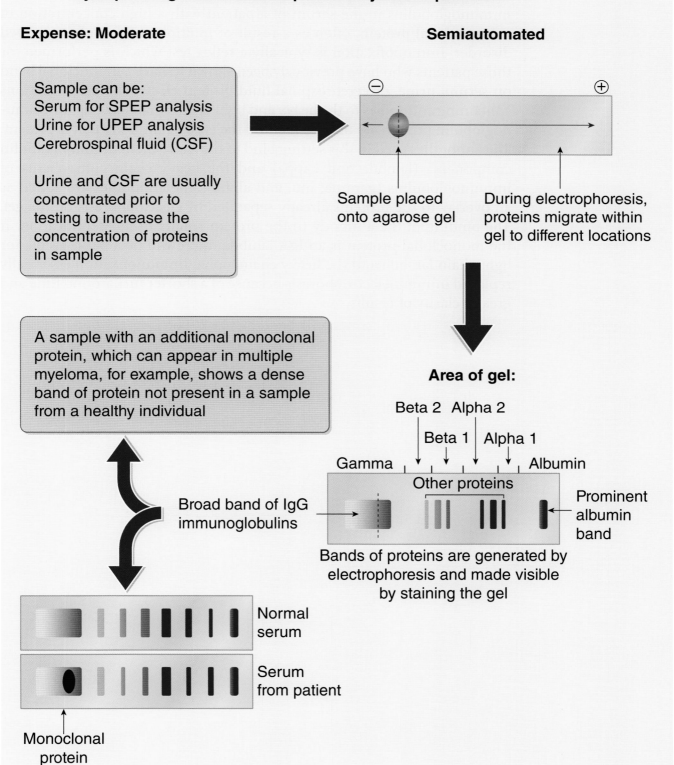

Expense: Moderate

Sample can be:
Serum for SPEP analysis
Urine for UPEP analysis
Cerebrospinal fluid (CSF)

Urine and CSF are usually concentrated prior to testing to increase the concentration of proteins in sample

Semiautomated

Sample placed onto agarose gel

During electrophoresis, proteins migrate within gel to different locations

A sample with an additional monoclonal protein, which can appear in multiple myeloma, for example, shows a dense band of protein not present in a sample from a healthy individual

Area of gel:

Beta 2   Alpha 2
Beta 1 | Alpha 1
Gamma   Albumin
Other proteins

Broad band of IgG immunoglobulins

Prominent albumin band

Bands of proteins are generated by electrophoresis and made visible by staining the gel

Normal serum

Serum from patient

Monoclonal protein

IMMUNOFIXATION TO IDENTIFY MONOCLONAL IMMUNOGLOBULINS

Immunofixation can identify proteins through the use of antibodies which bind to specific proteins. A common use is to identify monoclonal immunoglobulins in the serum of a patient with a high concentration of a monoclonal protein, often as a result of multiple myeloma or a related disorder. Immunofixation is typically a reflex test which is performed for those patients who have previously been shown to have a monoclonal band on serum, urine, or cerebrospinal fluid protein electrophoresis. Solutions containing antibodies to the heavy and light chains that make up the immunoglobulin protein are used to identify the type of antibody that is present. The antibodies used in this setting bind to the short chain immunoglobulin components (lambda and kappa) and the heavy chain components of immunoglobulins (gamma, mu, and alpha). The antibodies are added as an overlay to the proteins already separated by electrophoresis on the gel. The binding of the antibody to the protein results in its identification. If the monoclonal protein is an IgA lambda, there will be a band visible for light chain lambda and the heavy chain alpha. Immunofixation essentially replaced immunoelectrophoresis because of a shorter turnaround time and greater clarity of results.

Immunofixation to identify monoclonal immunoglobulins

To identify the heavy chain and the light chain in a monoclonal immunoglobulin by determining the antibodies which bind to the monoclonal protein

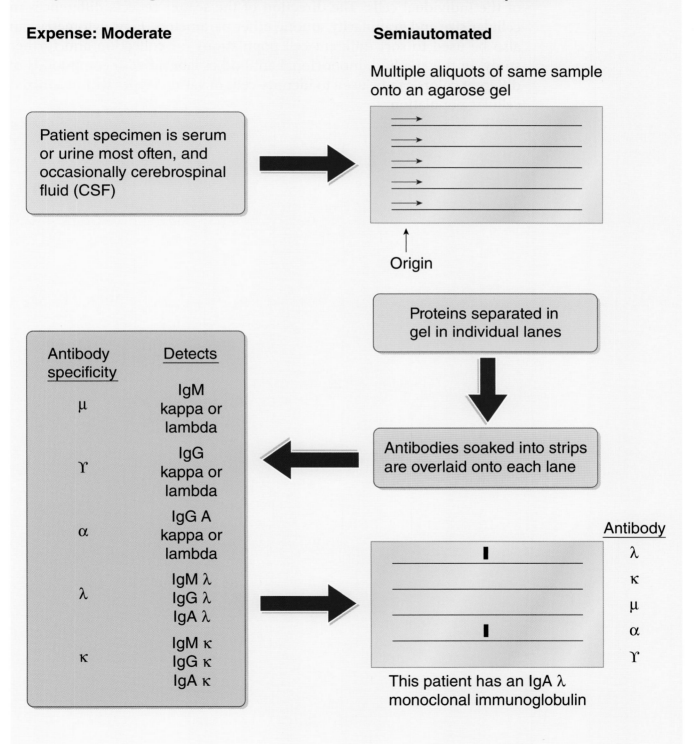

Expense: Moderate

Semiautomated

Patient specimen is serum or urine most often, and occasionally cerebrospinal fluid (CSF)

Multiple aliquots of same sample onto an agarose gel

Origin

Proteins separated in gel in individual lanes

Antibodies soaked into strips are overlaid onto each lane

Antibody specificity	Detects
μ	IgM kappa or lambda
Υ	IgG kappa or lambda
α	IgG A kappa or lambda
λ	IgM λ IgG λ IgA λ
κ	IgM κ IgG κ IgA κ

Antibody
λ
κ
μ
α
Υ

This patient has an IgA λ monoclonal immunoglobulin

FLOW CYTOMETRY

Flow cytometry is used to identify and count individual cells. Single cells are characterized by size, shape, and biochemical or antigenic composition. The cells flow in a single stream through a channel where they are exposed to a beam of light, which is scattered in all directions by the characteristics of the individual cells. The direction of the scatter reflects differences in cellular size and granularity, among other parameters. Flow cytometry can also be used to sort different cell populations for collection and further study. In this method, monoclonal antibodies labeled with compounds of different colors can be used to identify cells of various types within a mixed cellular population.

Flow cytometry

To identify cell type and assess cell surface markers through the use of antigen-specific fluorescent antibodies

Expense: High

Much manual processing with moderately complex instrumentation

For identification of cell type

For assessment of cell surface markers

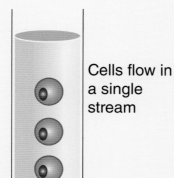

Cells flow in a single stream

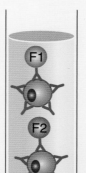

Cell suspension mixed with antibodies to different cell surface markers— each of which has a unique fluorescent label (F1 is different from F2)

Laser beam of light onto cell

From amount of light scattered forward and to the side, cell size, shape, and granularity determined— leading to identification of cell type

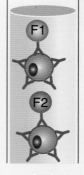

As cells flow in a stream within the instrument and are exposed to laser light, each fluorescent compound can be identified—fluorescent cells are positive for the cell surface marker with the specific fluorescent antibody to that surface marker

CRYOGLOBULIN ANALYSIS

Proteins known as cryoglobulins precipitate from plasma when the temperature of the plasma falls below 37 °C. Some cryoglobulins precipitate out at temperatures just below 37 °C. After separation of the serum from the blood cells by centrifugation, the tubes with serum being tested for cryoglobulins are refrigerated at 4 °C for 72 hours. At 24-hour intervals, the tubes are checked for formation of a precipitate. The amount of precipitate is quantitated, and the contents of the precipitate are evaluated electrophoretically to determine if the antibodies in the precipitate are monoclonal, mixed monoclonal and polyclonal, or mixed polyclonal.

Cryoglobulin analysis

To identify the type of proteins which precipitate out of serum and which suggest the presence of selected disorders

Expense: Moderate

Highly manual method

Cryoglobulins are proteins which precipitate out of serum at a temperature < 37 °C

37 °C

Therefore, all specimen transport and processing steps *must* be performed at 37 °C or the cryoglobulin may precipitate out of serum unintentionally prior to analysis

< 37 °C

◀—— Cryoprecipitate

Patient serum at 37 °C

➡

Sample split into 2 separate tubes and both placed at 4° for 1–3 days

Cryoglobulin in this tube processed by electrophoresis

Tube used to measure a packed "cryocrit" at 72 hours

Monoclonal immunoglobulins only
Cryoglobulinemia type I

Mixed monoclonal and polyclonal immunoglobulins
Cryoglobulinemia type II

Polyclonal immunoglobulins only
Cryoglobulinemia type III

2 Methods in Clinical Microbiology

GRAM STAIN

The Gram stain is used to rapidly identify organisms in a patient specimen and classify them as either gram-positive or gram-negative. This assay can identify in minutes a pathogenic organism if it is present in sufficient number and the test is performed correctly. This test requires microscopic examination of a stained slide, and recognition that gram-positive organisms are purple and gram-negative organisms are red. The specimen from a patient which may contain pathogenic organisms is applied to a glass slide, and then fixed and stained in a series of steps that ultimately leads to the differential staining of gram-positive and gram-negative organisms.

Gram stain

To identify infectious organisms in many different sample types by fixing and staining the organisms and examining the material on a glass side microscopically

Expense: Low

Manual with microscopic analysis required

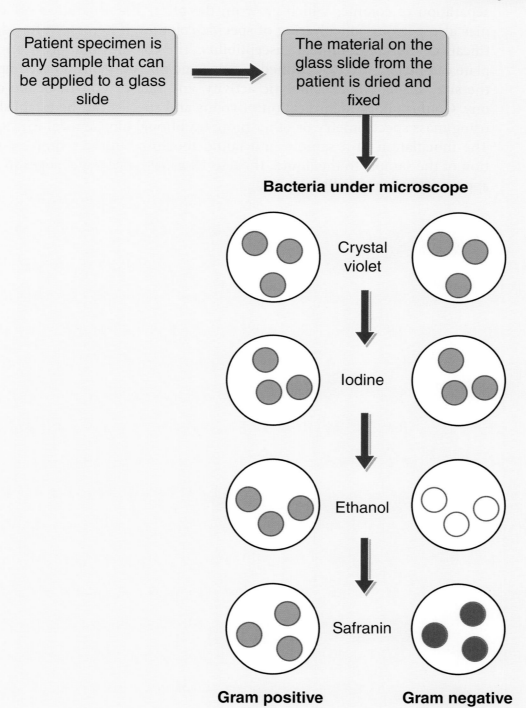

Patient specimen is any sample that can be applied to a glass slide

The material on the glass slide from the patient is dried and fixed

Bacteria under microscope

Crystal violet

Iodine

Ethanol

Safranin

Gram positive

Gram negative

MICROBIOLOGIC CULTURE AND ORGANISM IDENTIFICATION

Plating a microbiologic specimen from any of a variety of sites with a potential infection involves placement of the sample onto a bacteriologic plate containing solid medium or into a liquid medium that enhances bacteriologic growth. When applying a sample onto solid culture medium, the initial sample is spread onto the plate in a specific way to improve the separation of colonies which grow on the plate. The separation of colonies also permits subculturing of specific colonies, if necessary, for identification and antimicrobial susceptibility. The colonies that grow on the plate can be tentatively identified as a specific microorganism based upon the size, shape, color, hemolytic activity, and rate of growth of the colony. Confirmatory identification of genus and species can be established using mass spectrometry or other more traditional biochemical methods. The inoculation of a sample into liquid medium simply requires addition of the sample to the liquid. If bacterial growth occurs, changes in the appearance of the medium occur.

Microbiologic culture and organism identification

To identify pathogenic organisms by growing them in culture and assessing them after isolation with biochemical tests

Expense: Moderate to high, depending on the extent of the evaluation

Mostly manual with much visual inspection of colonies in different culture media

Sample collection	The sample to be processed can be:		
	Liquid—such as body fluids other than blood, which is processed differently	Solid or semisolid— such as sputum, stool, or tissue	On a swab from an infected site— such as a wound

Growth of organisms— in aerobic or anaerobic environments	The sample can be: Plated onto ≥1 agar plate to permit organisms to grow into colonies	Inoculated into a broth which promotes growth of microorganisms	Inoculated onto agar within a tube which promotes the growth of certain bacteria

Isolation of organisms	Colonies growing on agar surfaces are first characterized by colony morphology which provides an early clue to organism identification—and then colonies of interest can be subcultured for species identification

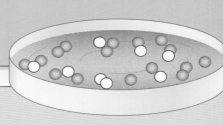

Identification of organisms	Microorganisms originating from an isolated colony can be tested in a panel of biochemical tests—the results of which identify the microorganism with a percent likelihood

BLOOD CULTURES

There is great concern for the presence of a pathogen in the circulating blood because sepsis is associated with high mortality. Blood samples are collected into specific bottles which promote the growth of microorganisms either aerobically or anaerobically. A specific amount of blood is added to a blood culture bottle immediately after the blood is collected in such a way that contamination with organisms from the skin or other site does not occur. The bottles are then placed in a specially equipped incubator which detects carbon dioxide generated within individual blood culture bottles. A positive blood culture is identified when there is generation of carbon dioxide associated with the growth of microorganisms. When a blood culture bottle becomes positive, it is then processed for identification of the microorganism and assessment of its antimicrobial sensitivity.

Blood cultures

To determine if there are infectious agents in the blood by promoting their growth in special medium and detecting their presence by CO_2 production

Expense: High   **In most laboratories it is now highly automated**

| Sample collection | The surface of the arm overlying the venipuncture site must be meticulously cleaned with agents that eliminate skin microorganisms before venipuncture—if not, non-pathogenic skin bacteria can contaminate the blood culture

Blood with or without microorganisms is collected into bottles for growth in aerobic or anaerobic environments |
|---|---|

Growth of organisms	Bottles are placed into specially equipped incubator for detection of carbon dioxide generated within individual blood culture bottles

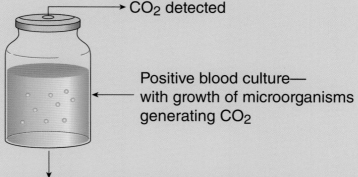

CO_2 detected

Positive blood culture— with growth of microorganisms generating CO_2

Sample from positive blood culture bottle is then processed for organism isolation, identification, and antimicrobial sensitivity

ANTIMICROBIAL SENSITIVITY TESTS

In the version of the assay called the dilution method, increasing concentrations of antimicrobial agents are added to separate tubes. Then a small volume of organism suspension is added to each tube, and the tubes are incubated and examined after a fixed period of time for bacterial growth. The tube with the lowest antibiotic concentration which shows no bacterial growth identifies what is known as the minimal inhibitory concentration (MIC) for that antimicrobial agent against that organism.

In a less commonly used method, known as the disk diffusion method, a suspension of organisms is distributed over the surface of a culture plate, and then disks which contain different antimicrobial agents are dropped onto the plate. The plate is incubated for a fixed period of time, and if the pathogen is susceptible to the antimicrobial agent, there will be a zone of inhibition around the desk. The larger the zone of inhibition, the more susceptible the organism is to treatment with that particular antibiotic in the disk.

Antimicrobial sensitivity tests

To determine which antibiotics are likely to effectively eliminate an infectious organism by exposing the organism to different antibiotics in vitro

Expense: High

Can be highly manual, as in disc diffusion method, or semiautomated, as in dilution method

Microorganisms originating from an isolated colony are placed in a liquid suspension

Dilution method

Organisms into multiple tubes

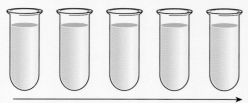

More antimicrobial agent into each sequential tube

After incubation, concentration of antimicrobial agent that inhibits organism growth is determined

Minimum inhibitory drug concentration

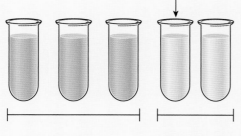

Organisms growing   Organisms not growing

Disc diffusion method

Organisms spread to completely cover a large agar plate which supports organism growth

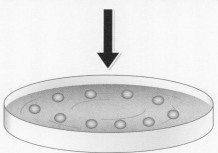

Discs with different antimicrobial agents placed onto agar surface and drug slowly diffuses from disc

After incubation, agents which inhibit growth of organisms are identified because bacterial growth is far from the disc

Organism-free zone

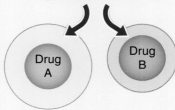

Drug A is a better antimicrobial agent than drug B

DIRECT AND INDIRECT IMMUNOFLUORESCENCE FOR ANTIGEN DETECTION

These tests can demonstrate the presence of a specific antigen or an antibody to a specific antigen in a specimen. The patient's specimen is applied onto a glass slide. In the direct immunofluorescence test, a fluorescent-labeled antibody to the antigen of interest is layered onto the glass slide to which the patient's sample is bound. Fluorescence indicates the presence of the antigen of interest. In the indirect test, antibodies against the antigen of interest are detected. To perform this assay, an antibody which specifically detects an antigen of interest is layered onto the glass slide. Then, a fluorescent-labeled antihuman IgG antibody is added onto the glass slide. The second antibody detects antibodies in the patient's sample which have become bound to an antigen of interest.

Direct and indirect immunofluorescence for antigen detection

To assess for a variety of specific antigens by using antibodies to the antigens with detection by fluorescence in a microscopic examination

Expense: Moderate   **Manual with microscopic evaluation**

Direct immunofluorescence

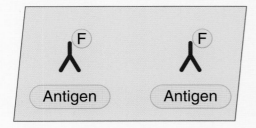

Fluorescent F labeled antibody binds to antigen of interest on a glass slide or other surface

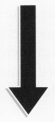

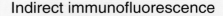
Indirect immunofluorescence

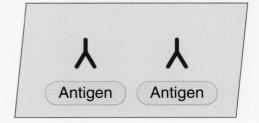

Antibody which is *not* fluorescent-labeled binds to antigen of interest on a glass slide or other surface

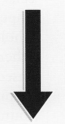

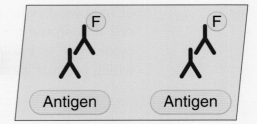

Slides read using a fluorescent microscope

Fluorescent F labeled antibody to IgG is added and binds to antibody previously bound to antigen

3

Methods in Clinical Hematology

COUNTING OF BLOOD CELLS WITH AUTOMATED WHITE BLOOD CELL DIFFERENTIAL COUNT

In most automated instruments that count cells in the blood, the red blood cells, the white blood cells, and the platelets are counted by an electrical impedance method. In addition, hemoglobin is measured directly from the whole blood specimen after lysis of the red blood cells. There are many other parameters in an automated blood cell count, which are calculated, based upon the data obtained from the direct cell counts and the hemoglobin value. Calculated parameters include the hematocrit, red blood cell count, the mean corpuscular volume (MCV), the mean corpuscular hemoglobin (MCH), the mean corpuscular hemoglobin concentration (MCHC) of red blood cells, and the mean platelet volume (MPV). The white blood cell differential count is obtained after lysis of erythrocytes, using flow cytometric technology to identify size, shape, and granularity of the cells which permits identification of the individual white blood cell populations.

Counting of blood cells with automated white blood cell differential count

To enumerate the number of white blood cells and the major white blood cell types; the number of red blood cells by cell counting and hemoglobin analysis, along with determination of red blood cell indices; and the number of platelets

Expense: Low   **Highly automated**

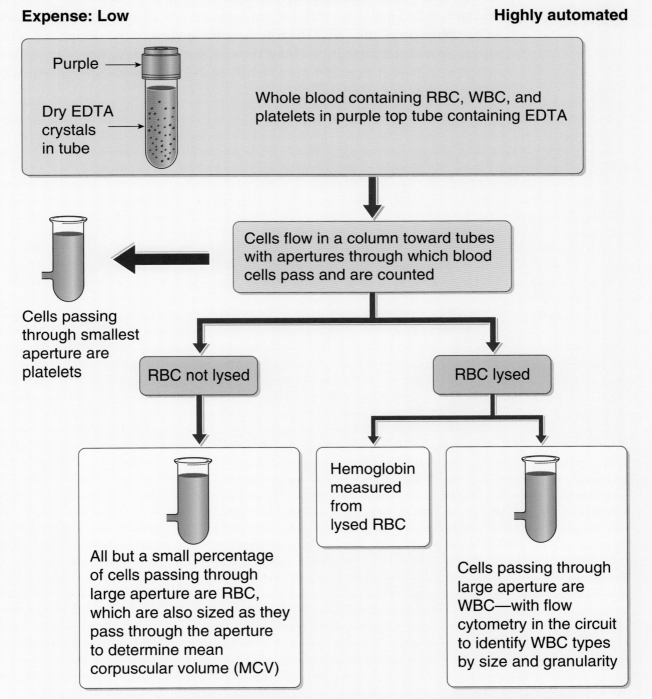

Purple

Dry EDTA crystals in tube

Whole blood containing RBC, WBC, and platelets in purple top tube containing EDTA

Cells flow in a column toward tubes with apertures through which blood cells pass and are counted

Cells passing through smallest aperture are platelets

RBC not lysed

RBC lysed

Hemoglobin measured from lysed RBC

All but a small percentage of cells passing through large aperture are RBC, which are also sized as they pass through the aperture to determine mean corpuscular volume (MCV)

Cells passing through large aperture are WBC—with flow cytometry in the circuit to identify WBC types by size and granularity

Hematocrit or packed RBC volume is calculated from number and size of RBC

PERIPHERAL BLOOD SMEAR ANALYSIS

A peripheral blood smear is prepared by adding a drop of blood to a glass slide and smearing it in a specific way to spread out the blood cells for microscopic examination. Most commonly, a small device spreads the drop of blood on the surface. The sample is stained with Wright stain, and the smear is then reviewed microscopically at low and high magnification. Certain cells tend aggregate along the edges of the smear. There is a recommended procedure for microscopic review to account for variability in distribution of the cells. The microscopic review of the peripheral blood smear provides information about the size, shape, and number of red blood cells, the different populations of white blood cells, and an approximation of the number of platelets.

Peripheral blood smear analysis

To determine the size, shape, and any abnormal morphology of all blood cell types by examining a stained preparation of blood cells microscopically

Expense: Low

Smear preparation automated or manual, followed by microscopic examination

Sample collected into a purple top tube containing EDTA

Drop of blood is applied to a glass slide and smeared to spread blood cells across slide

Drop of blood →

Smeared blood on slide

Microscopic examination is performed to detect abnormalities in number or in appearance of:

Red blood cells

White blood cells

Platelets

The peripheral blood smear is commonly used early in the diagnostic process to assess a patient for an abnormality involving circulating blood cells

SICKLE CELL SCREENING ASSAY

This test provides a rapid assessment for the presence of hemoglobin S. Further analysis of different hemoglobin types is performed by hemoglobin analysis. In one commonly used test called the sickling test, a drop of the patient's blood is placed onto a glass slide, and a reducing agent or normal saline (as a control) is added to the drop of blood on the slide. If sickle hemoglobin is present, the red blood cells from the patient exposed to the reducing agent show sickling.

In the solubility test, a reducing agent is added to a tube containing the patient's blood. After incubation, the tube is placed in front of a card with black lines. The solubility test is positive for sickle hemoglobin when black lines cannot be seen through the specimen. The solution is turbid as a result of insoluble crystals of hemoglobin S.

Sickle cell screening assay

To rapidly assess for the presence of hemoglobin S by using methods involving either predisposition of red blood cells to sickle or the limited solubility of hemoglobin S.

Expense: Moderate

Manual assays, and the sickling test requires microscopic examination

Sample of blood collected into purple top tube containing EDTA—two available tests to detect sickle hemoglobin illustrated here

Sickling test—
Blood onto glass slide, followed by addition of reducing agent over blood droplet

Solubility test—
Blood added to a concentrated phosphate buffer solution, followed by RBC lytic agent and reducing agent

Hemoglobin S detected by presence of holly leaf or sickle cells upon microscopic exam

Hemoglobin S detected if buffer becomes turbid because hemoglobin S is not soluble in this buffer

Tests are positive for patients with:
Hemoglobin SS (sickle cell anemia)
Hemoglobin AS (sickle trait)
Hemoglobin S with another abnormal hemoglobin (example: hemoglobin SC)

  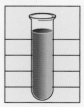 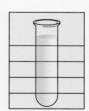

RBC with normal morphology

RBC with abnormal morphology after addition of reducing agent

Turbid solution
Positive

Clear solution
Negative

HEMOGLOBIN ANALYSIS

Many different hemoglobins have arisen through alterations in the genes that code for alpha and beta globin. The appropriate treatment of patients with an abnormal hemoglobin requires identification of the specific hemoglobin which is present. To identify the different hemoglobins present in a patient's red blood cells, the red blood cells are first isolated from whole blood. Red blood cells are then hemolyzed, and it is this hemolysate that is the starting material for hemoglobin analysis. The different types of hemoglobin can be separated by a variety of different techniques. Commonly used separation techniques include gel electrophoresis, high-performance liquid chromatography, and isoelectric focusing.

Hemoglobin analysis

To determine the different hemoglobins present by one or more methods which separate hemoglobin types

Expense: Moderate   **Semiautomated**

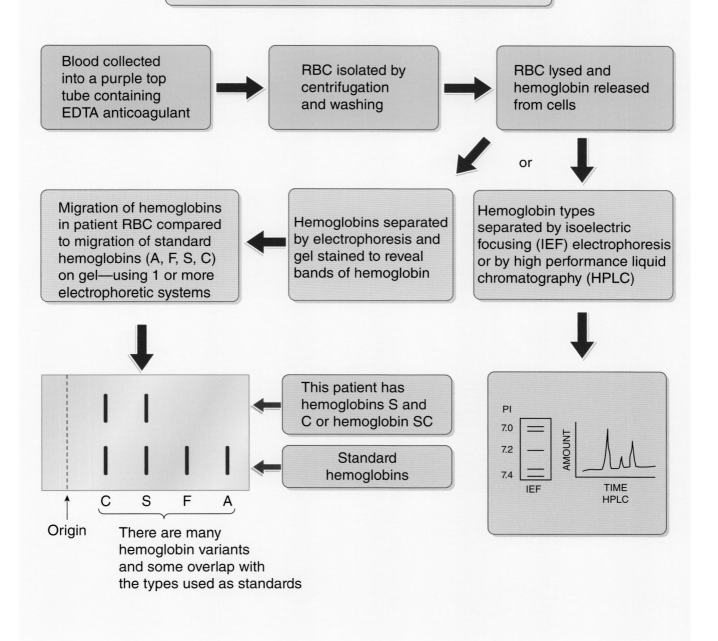

Goal of the test is to identify the hemoglobin types present in a patient's red blood cells (RBC)

Blood collected into a purple top tube containing EDTA anticoagulant

RBC isolated by centrifugation and washing

RBC lysed and hemoglobin released from cells

or

Migration of hemoglobins in patient RBC compared to migration of standard hemoglobins (A, F, S, C) on gel—using 1 or more electrophoretic systems

Hemoglobins separated by electrophoresis and gel stained to reveal bands of hemoglobin

Hemoglobin types separated by isoelectric focusing (IEF) electrophoresis or by high performance liquid chromatography (HPLC)

This patient has hemoglobins S and C or hemoglobin SC

Standard hemoglobins

C   S   F   A

Origin

There are many hemoglobin variants and some overlap with the types used as standards

PI
7.0
7.2
7.4
IEF

AMOUNT

TIME
HPLC

ERYTHROCYTE SEDIMENTATION RATE

The erythrocyte sedimentation rate (ESR), a general assessment for inflammation, measures the decrease in the height of a layer of red blood cells within a long slender tube after a fixed period of time. The number of millimeters the column of red cells settles over this time is the ESR. There are multiple variations of this test to optimize its performance. C-reactive protein is also a general assessment for inflammation, and it is measured by other methods.

Erythrocyte sedimentation rate and C-Reactive Protein Measurement

To assess systemic inflammation by measuring the extent of red blood cell sedimentation over a fixed period of time or the amount of C-Reactive Protein in the plasma or serum

Expense: Low   **Manual or semiautomated**

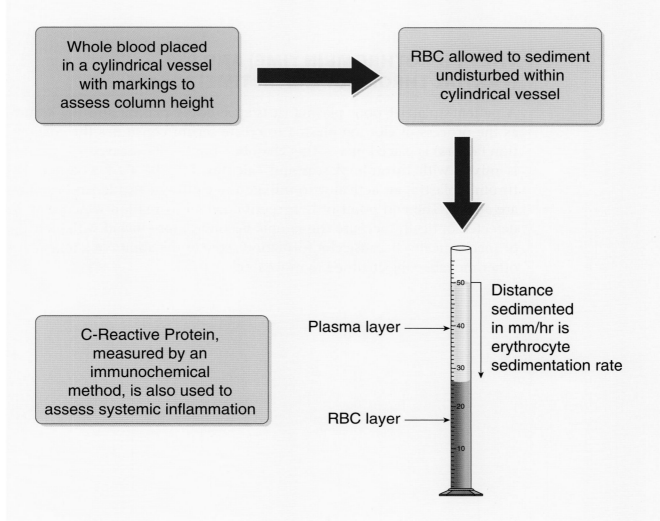

Goal of the test is to measure the height of sedimented RBC after an incubation, often 1 hour

Whole blood placed in a cylindrical vessel with markings to assess column height

RBC allowed to sediment undisturbed within cylindrical vessel

C-Reactive Protein, measured by an immunochemical method, is also used to assess systemic inflammation

Plasma layer — 40

RBC layer — 20

Distance sedimented in mm/hr is erythrocyte sedimentation rate

4 Methods in Clinical Coagulation

THE PT (PROTHROMBIN TIME) AND PTT (PARTIAL THROMBOPLASTIN TIME) ASSAYS

A patient's platelet-poor plasma (it is specifically plasma and not serum, as the process of clotting plasma to create serum consumes the coagulation factors) is placed in a testing chamber. For the PT assay, the specimen is mixed with thromboplastin and calcium. For the PTT assay, partial thromboplastin, an activator to initiate the clotting cascade, and calcium are added. The end point of the reaction is clot formation which may be detected optically, because the sample becomes more turbid with clotting, or mechanically, because clot formation reduces the ability of a magnet or other movable object added to move freely.

The PT and PTT assays

To assess the amount of coagulation factor activity by measuring the time to clot formation after adding agents to activate the coagulation cascade

Expense: Low   **Highly automated**

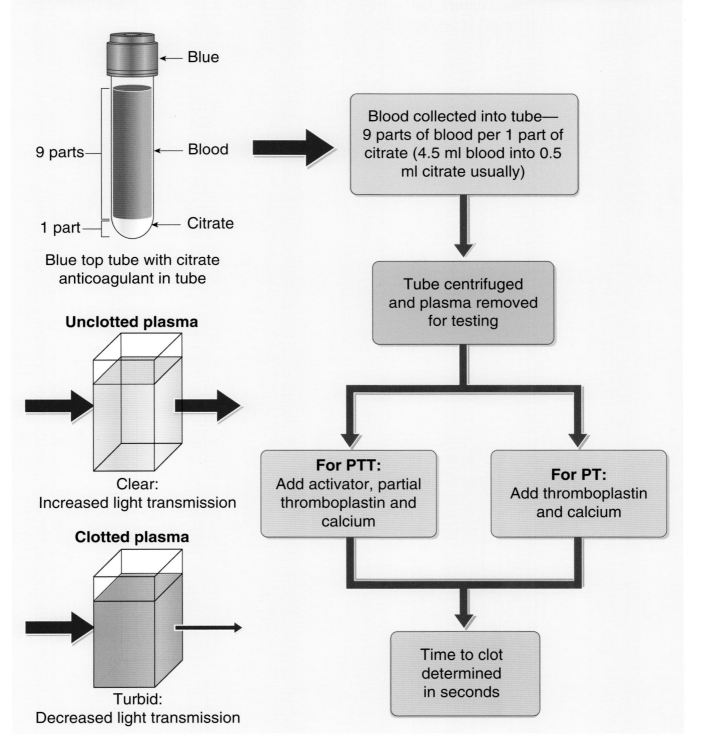

Blue ←

9 parts ← Blood

1 part ← Citrate

Blue top tube with citrate anticoagulant in tube

Unclotted plasma

Clear: Increased light transmission

Clotted plasma

Turbid: Decreased light transmission

Blood collected into tube— 9 parts of blood per 1 part of citrate (4.5 ml blood into 0.5 ml citrate usually)

Tube centrifuged and plasma removed for testing

For PTT: Add activator, partial thromboplastin and calcium

For PT: Add thromboplastin and calcium

Time to clot determined in seconds

PT AND PTT MIXING STUDIES

To determine if an elevated value for the PT or the PTT is the result of an inhibitor or one or more factor deficiencies, a sample of the patient plasma is mixed in equal parts with a sample of normal plasma. The mixed plasma is then placed at 37 °C immediately after mixing, and then again at 30, 60, and, if desired, 120 minutes of incubation, a sample is removed from the mixture, and a PT or PTT (whichever is elevated above the reference range) is performed.

PT and PTT mixing studies

To determine if a prolonged PT or prolonged PTT is a result of a coagulation factor deficiency or an inhibitor that affects the coagulation cascade, by measuring the time to clot formation using the patient plasma after it is mixed in equal parts with normal plasma

Expense: Low

After samples are mixed, the testing is highly automated

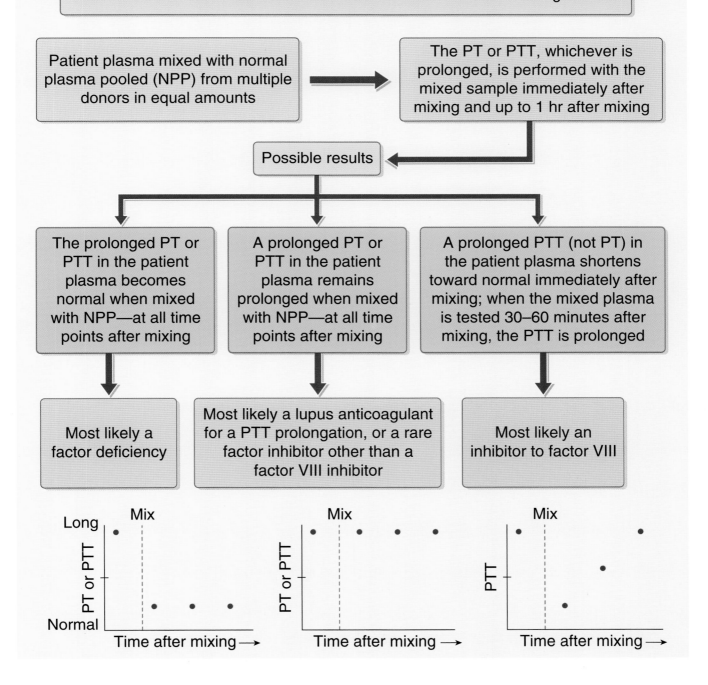

The goal of the test is to determine if a prolonged PT or prolonged PTT is a result of ≥1 factor deficiencies or an inhibitor of the PT or PTT clotting reaction

Patient plasma mixed with normal plasma pooled (NPP) from multiple donors in equal amounts

The PT or PTT, whichever is prolonged, is performed with the mixed sample immediately after mixing and up to 1 hr after mixing

Possible results

The prolonged PT or PTT in the patient plasma becomes normal when mixed with NPP—at all time points after mixing

A prolonged PT or PTT in the patient plasma remains prolonged when mixed with NPP—at all time points after mixing

A prolonged PTT (not PT) in the patient plasma shortens toward normal immediately after mixing; when the mixed plasma is tested 30–60 minutes after mixing, the PTT is prolonged

Most likely a factor deficiency

Most likely a lupus anticoagulant for a PTT prolongation, or a rare factor inhibitor other than a factor VIII inhibitor

Most likely an inhibitor to factor VIII

COAGULATION FACTOR ASSAYS

To measure the amount of an individual coagulation factor, the test is a modified PT or PTT. The patient's plasma is mixed with plasma deficient in the single factor being assayed. In this way, the patient's plasma is the only source of the coagulation factor which is present in the sample. Coagulation factor assays are based upon the PT (adding thromboplastin and calcium) for factors II, V, VII, and X; or the PTT (adding partial thromboplastin, an activator of the coagulation cascade, and calcium) for factors VIII, IX, XI, and XII.

Coagulation factor assays

To quantitate the amount of a specific coagulation factor by determining the time to clot formation using the patient plasma mixed with plasma deficient only in the coagulation factor being measured

Expense: Moderate, due to reagents used

Highly automated after dilution and mixing steps

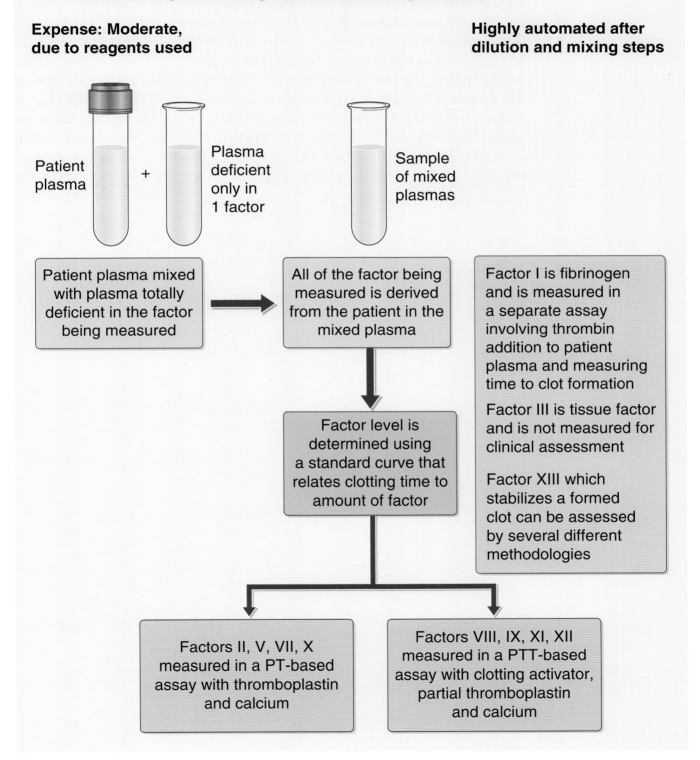

Patient plasma + Plasma deficient only in 1 factor

Sample of mixed plasmas

Patient plasma mixed with plasma totally deficient in the factor being measured

All of the factor being measured is derived from the patient in the mixed plasma

Factor I is fibrinogen and is measured in a separate assay involving thrombin addition to patient plasma and measuring time to clot formation

Factor III is tissue factor and is not measured for clinical assessment

Factor XIII which stabilizes a formed clot can be assessed by several different methodologies

Factor level is determined using a standard curve that relates clotting time to amount of factor

Factors II, V, VII, X measured in a PT-based assay with thromboplastin and calcium

Factors VIII, IX, XI, XII measured in a PTT-based assay with clotting activator, partial thromboplastin and calcium

VON WILLEBRAND FACTOR ASSAYS

There are now several different assays to assess the function of von Willebrand factor. The ristocetin cofactor assay has been the primary method to measure von Willebrand factor activity for decades. It is now being replaced with a variety of assays using different methodologies (not shown here), and the need for a replacement is driven by the high complexity and imprecision of the ristocetin cofactor test. There is no dominant assay in use currently. Ristocetin cofactor is the name given to the test because ristocetin is the principal reagent in this assay. Using formalin-fixed platelets, the rate of platelet aggregation upon addition of ristocetin to the sample is measured to provide a quantitative value for von Willebrand factor function. It is important to note that it is not the plateau value for platelet aggregation that is related to the activity of von Willebrand factor. Instead it is the rate at which the platelets aggregate, as determined from the slope of the line in the platelet aggregation tracing.

von Willebrand factor assays

To measure the activity of von Willebrand factor by measuring the ability of von Willebrand factor to promote platelet aggregation; and to measure the amount of von Willebrand protein using an immunoassay.

Expense: High

Test for ristocetin cofactor is largely manual, and tests for von Willebrand factor antigen can be semiautomated

Test for von Willebrand factor function: the ristocetin cofactor assay (One of the several tests to measure von Willebrand factor function)

Test to assess the amount of von Willebrand factor protein: the von Willebrand antigen assay

The amount of von Willebrand factor activity is proportional to the rate at which fixed platelets aggregate in response to ristocetin

Enzyme-linked immunoassay (ELISA) and other methods involving antibody to von Willebrand factor can be used to quantify amount of von Willebrand factor protein

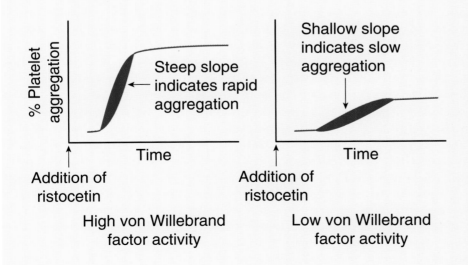

PLATELET AGGREGATION

There are many tests used to assess the function of platelets. The "gold standard" test for platelet function is the one that assesses the ability of platelets to aggregate in response to agonists which activate platelets. The test is performed in a specialized instrument called an aggregometer. The sample used for analysis is platelet-rich plasma. The plasma-containing platelets are added to different cuvettes, and then platelet activators are added to the individual cuvettes. Detection of aggregation is measured as the large platelet clumps fall to the bottom, producing an increase in the transmission of light through the sample in the cuvette.

Platelet aggregation

To determine the function of platelets by assessing their ability to aggregate when exposed to platelet activating agents

Expense: High

Manual test requiring careful performance to generate accurate result

Goal of the test is to assess the function of circulating platelets

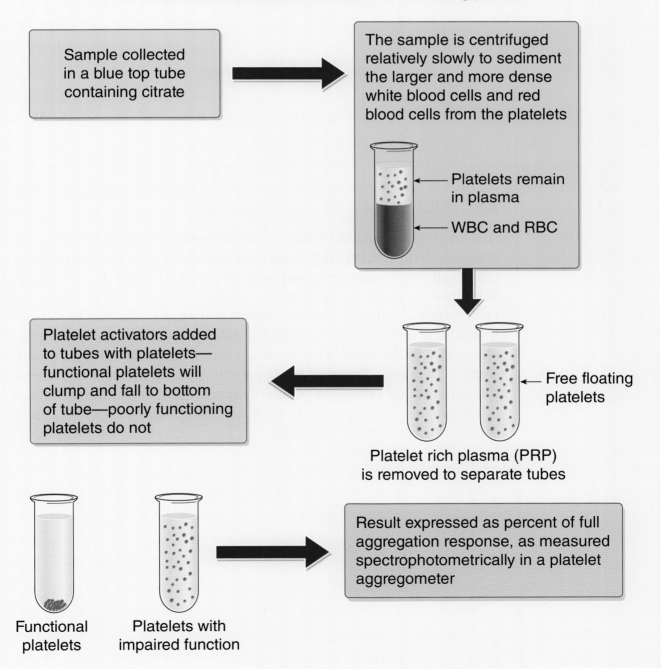

Sample collected in a blue top tube containing citrate

The sample is centrifuged relatively slowly to sediment the larger and more dense white blood cells and red blood cells from the platelets

Platelets remain in plasma

WBC and RBC

Platelet activators added to tubes with platelets—functional platelets will clump and fall to bottom of tube—poorly functioning platelets do not

Free floating platelets

Platelet rich plasma (PRP) is removed to separate tubes

Functional platelets

Platelets with impaired function

Result expressed as percent of full aggregation response, as measured spectrophotometrically in a platelet aggregometer

5

Methods in Transfusion Medicine and Blood Banking

ABO/Rh TYPING

ABO typing of red blood cells is a two-step process. Forward typing detects antigens on the patient's red blood cells. Separate tubes with the patient's red blood cell suspension are mixed with a solution of antibodies against group A antigen, group B antigen, or Rh antigen. The presence of agglutination or hemolysis indicates that antibody has bound to the red blood cells in that tube, and that the antigen of interest is present. Reverse typing detects antibodies in the patient's plasma against antigens on the red blood cell surface. In reverse typing, it is the patient's plasma that is used rather than the patient's red cells. The plasma is mixed with cells known to have an A antigen or a B antigen. As in forward typing, agglutination or hemolysis indicates that antibody is present.

ABO/Rh typing

To determine the ABO blood type and Rh status by measuring the clumping of red blood cells after addition of antibodies to A, B, and Rh antigens; and by assessing for clumping of red blood cells known to have A or B surface antigens after addition of patient serum

Expense: Low   **Automated or manual**

Forward typing:
To detect antigens on RBC

Reverse typing:
To detect antibodies in serum which can bind to RBC antigens

Add antibodies to A, B, and Rh antigens in 3 separate tubes (1 for A, 1 for B, 1 for Rh) containing patient RBC

Add patient serum with or without anti-A and anti-B antibodies to A positive and to B positive RBC (A cells in 1 tube and B cells in another)

Clumping of RBC indicates presence of antigen on RBC

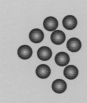

Failure to clump indicates absence of antigen on RBC

Clumping of RBC indicates presence of antibody to RBC antigen on cells used (either A or B)

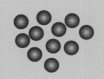

Failure to clump indicates absence of antibody to RBC antigen

BLOOD COMPONENT PREPARATION

Whole blood is collected from a donor into a bag which contains an anticoagulant that mixes with the blood as it enters the bag to prevent clotting. A predetermined weight of blood is collected. After sealing, the blood is first separated into red blood cells and platelet-rich plasma by centrifugation. The packed red blood cell component is then available for testing prior to transfusion. The platelet-rich plasma is transferred to a second bag, which is centrifuged to separate the plasma from the pellet of platelets. The plasma is removed from the platelets and is available for testing prior to freezing and subsequent transfusion. The platelets are resuspended to create a "random donor" platelet concentrate. "Single donor" platelets are collected by apheresis. In this way, packed red blood cells, fresh frozen plasma, and random donor platelet concentrates are prepared from a single unit of whole blood.

Blood component preparation

To produce packed red blood cells, fresh frozen plasma, platelet concentrates, and plasma-derived products including cryoprecipitate, immunoglobulins, albumin, and coagulation factor concentrates by different centrifugation and precipitation steps

Expense: Blood products are expensive; separation of whole blood into blood components is moderately expensive

The process of component preparation is manual

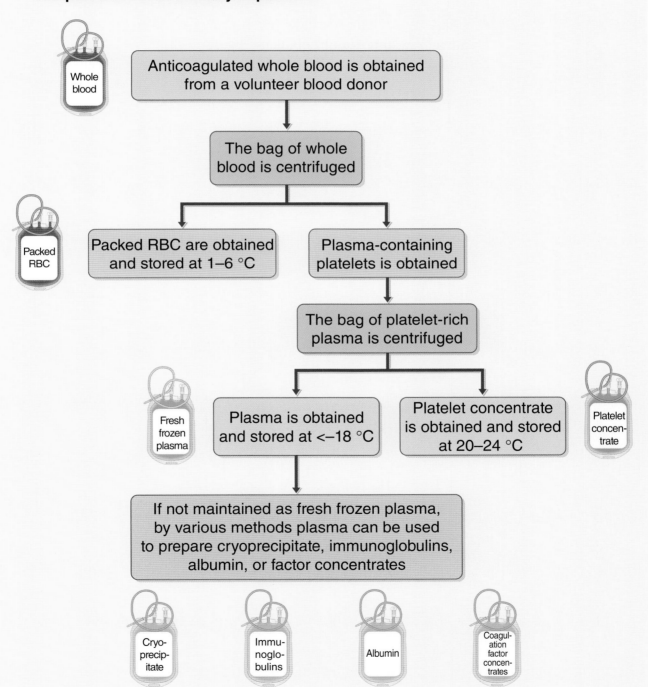

Whole blood

Anticoagulated whole blood is obtained from a volunteer blood donor

The bag of whole blood is centrifuged

Packed RBC

Packed RBC are obtained and stored at 1–6 °C

Plasma-containing platelets is obtained

The bag of platelet-rich plasma is centrifuged

Fresh frozen plasma

Plasma is obtained and stored at <–18 °C

Platelet concentrate is obtained and stored at 20–24 °C

Platelet concentrate

If not maintained as fresh frozen plasma, by various methods plasma can be used to prepare cryoprecipitate, immunoglobulins, albumin, or factor concentrates

Cryoprecipitate

Immunoglobulins

Albumin

Coagulation factor concentrates

BLOOD CROSSMATCH

The crossmatch test for ABO incompatibility identifies clinically significant patient antibodies to the red blood cells of a potential red blood cell donor. To identify antibodies to donor red blood cells, the patient's serum is mixed with a small volume of the donor's red blood cells, and the red blood cell suspension is then checked for agglutination or hemolysis. The presence of agglutination or hemolysis indicates that the cross match is incompatible, and that the tested donor unit is not suitable for transfusion.

Blood crossmatch

To determine the suitability of a donated packed red blood cell product for a potential recipient by assessing for donor red blood cell agglutination or hemolysis when mixed with serum from the potential recipient

Expense: Low   **Process described below is manual**

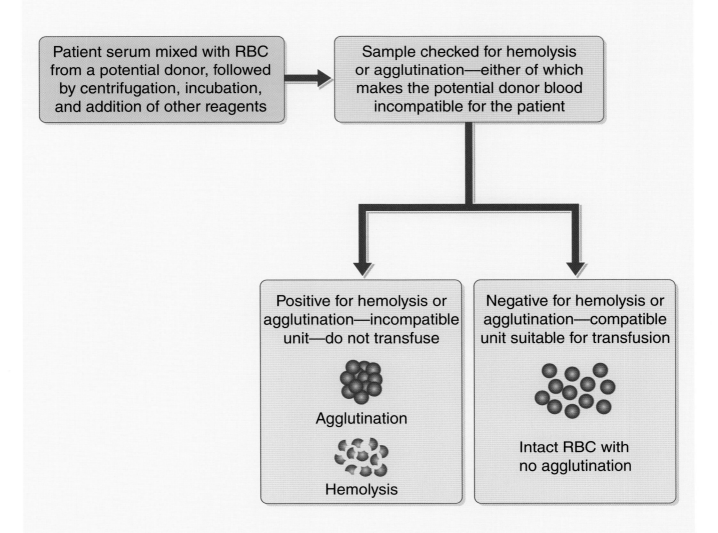

The goal of the test is to determine if anything in the blood of a patient recipient will hemolyze or agglutinate the RBC from a potential donor

Patient serum mixed with RBC from a potential donor, followed by centrifugation, incubation, and addition of other reagents

Sample checked for hemolysis or agglutination—either of which makes the potential donor blood incompatible for the patient

Positive for hemolysis or agglutination—incompatible unit—do not transfuse

Agglutination

Hemolysis

Negative for hemolysis or agglutination—compatible unit suitable for transfusion

Intact RBC with no agglutination

DIRECT ANTIGLOBULIN TEST (DAT)

To determine if a red blood cell has IgG immunoglobulin or the complement component C3d bound to its surface, a suspension of red blood cells from a patient is mixed with antibodies against IgG or C3d. If agglutination of the red cells is observed, the test is positive, indicating the presence of IgG or C3d on the surface of the red blood cells.

Direct antiglobulin test (DAT)

To determine if IgG or C3d is bound to the red blood cell surface by assessing for red blood cell clumping or hemolysis when the patient red cells are mixed with antibody to IgG or C3d

Expense: Moderate   **Largely manual method**

Goal of the test is to determine if IgG immunoglobin or C3d complement is bound to the surface of the patient's red blood cells

Suspension of patient's RBC placed in 3 separate tubes

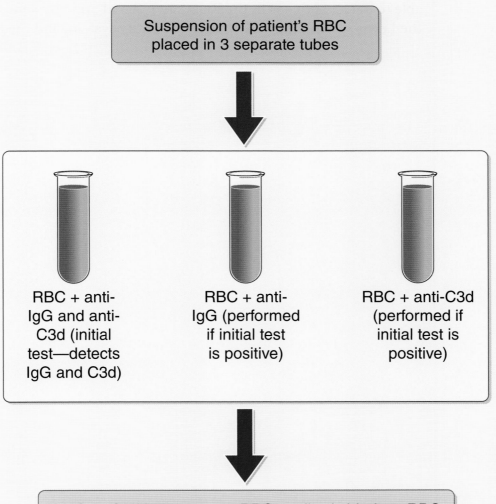

RBC + anti-IgG and anti-C3d (initial test—detects IgG and C3d)

RBC + anti-IgG (performed if initial test is positive)

RBC + anti-C3d (performed if initial test is positive)

If IgG or C3d is present on RBC, antibody binds to RBC, resulting in RBC agglutination and/or RBC hemolysis

INDIRECT ANTIGLOBULIN TEST (IAT)

The IAT detects antibodies to red blood cells which are present in a blood sample. The blood may be from a blood donor or from a potential recipient in need of a red blood cell transfusion. Red blood cells that express known antigens, called reagent cells, are the reagents used in this assay. If there is an antibody in the plasma or serum against an antigen on the different reagent cells, the antibodies will bind to the reagent red cells with that antigen and induce agglutination or hemolysis. A positive reaction with the reagent cells indicates that the plasma or serum sample tested has an antibody which binds to red blood cells with that antigen. A patient should not be transfused with red blood cells until the antigen specificity of the red blood cell antibody is known. Once the target antigen of the red blood cell antibody is known, only red blood cell components negative for the antigen are selected for transfusion. The different reagent cell types must be able to detect antigens in the Rh system, the M and S system, the P system, the Lewis system, the Kell system, the Duffy system, and the Kidd system.

Indirect antiglobulin test (IAT)

To detect antibodies in the plasma or serum that can become bound to red blood cells by assessing for red blood cell clumping or hemolysis when the patient plasma or serum is mixed with red blood cells that have specific known antigens

Expense: Moderate

Largely manual method

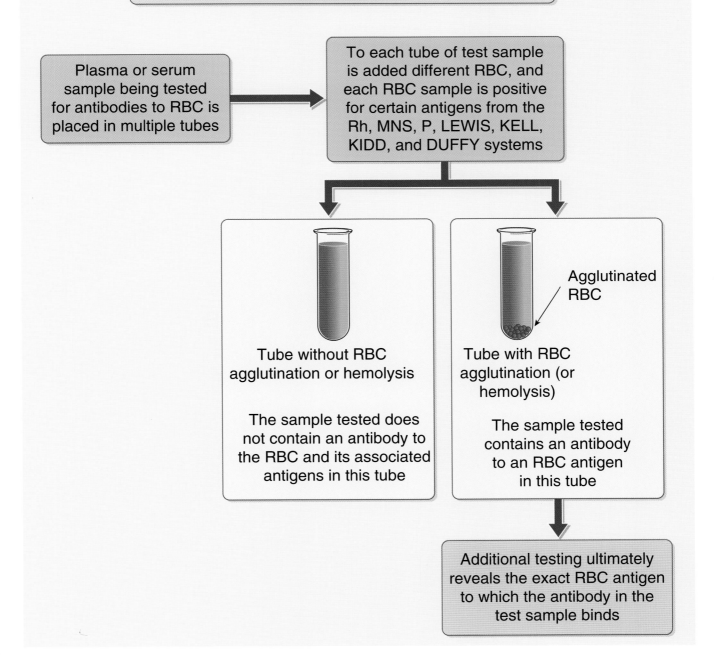

APHERESIS

Apheresis, more commonly called pheresis, is a process whereby a blood component is removed from the patient or donor while other blood components are returned. This may be plasmapheresis (removal of plasma), plateletpheresis (removal of platelets), leukapheresis (removal of white blood cells), or red blood cell exchange. In plasmapheresis, there is simultaneous replacement of blood with a colloid solution or normal plasma, depending upon the indication for the apheresis.

Apheresis

To remove plasma or specific blood cells from patients for therapeutic purposes; or to remove platelets from healthy donors for transfusion of patients who will benefit from an increase in platelet count

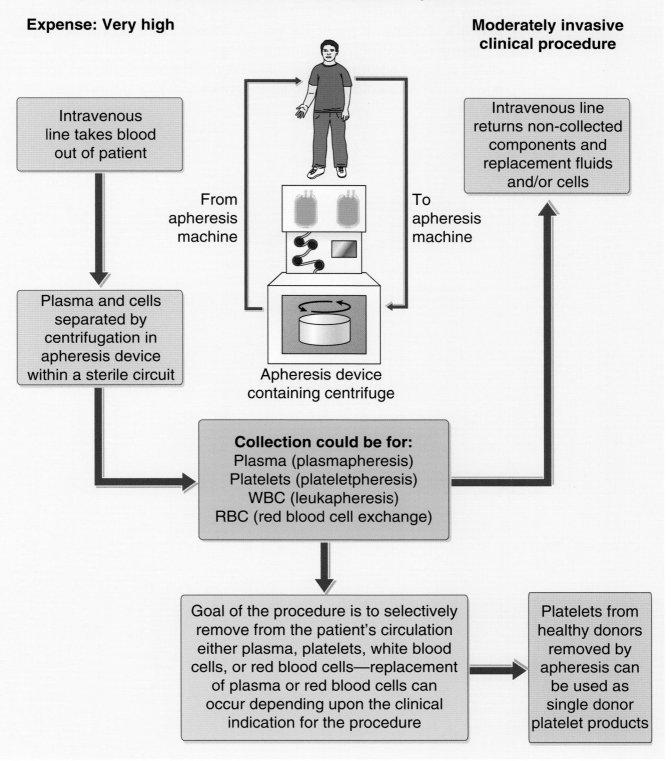

Expense: Very high

Moderately invasive clinical procedure

Intravenous line takes blood out of patient

From apheresis machine

To apheresis machine

Intravenous line returns non-collected components and replacement fluids and/or cells

Plasma and cells separated by centrifugation in apheresis device within a sterile circuit

Apheresis device containing centrifuge

Collection could be for:
Plasma (plasmapheresis)
Platelets (plateletpheresis)
WBC (leukapheresis)
RBC (red blood cell exchange)

Goal of the procedure is to selectively remove from the patient's circulation either plasma, platelets, white blood cells, or red blood cells—replacement of plasma or red blood cells can occur depending upon the clinical indication for the procedure

Platelets from healthy donors removed by apheresis can be used as single donor platelet products

WESTERN BLOT

This test is essentially identical to immunofixation electrophoresis. The first step involves preparation of a reagent strip on which a protein suspension is separated by electrophoresis. The strip with separated proteins is then incubated with patient's serum to determine if the sample contains antibodies to any of the proteins on the reagent strip. If there is an antibody in the patient's serum to a particular protein, those proteins will be identified following the addition of antihuman immunoglobulin conjugated with an enzyme. Upon addition of the substrate of the enzyme to which the antibody is linked, a colored product is generated which appears as a line on the gel.

Western blot

To identify antibodies in the blood of patients directed at specific proteins by binding to antigens fixed to a surface

Expense: High   **Manual method**

Goal is to identify antibodies in patient serum directed at specific proteins

Example: Identification of antibodies in serum to proteins within the human immunodeficiency virus (HIV)

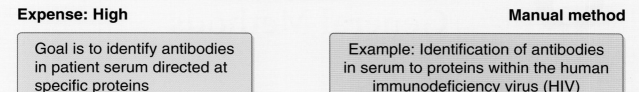

Proteins bound to solid phase—but not stained—no protein bands visible

If antibody is present which binds to this protein, it will bind

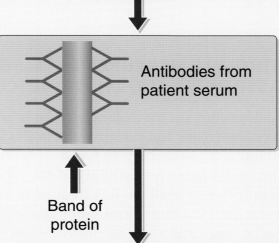

Antibodies from patient serum

Band of protein

Antibody binding detected by anti-human immunoglobulin linked to an enzyme E

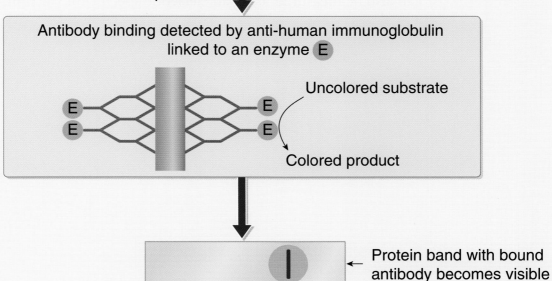

Uncolored substrate

Colored product

Protein band with bound antibody becomes visible

6 Methods in Clinical Chemistry and General Methods

ELECTROLYTE MEASUREMENTS: SODIUM (Na), POTASSIUM (K), AND CHLORIDE (Cl)

The concentrations of the major electrolytes in venous plasma or serum can be determined using ion-selective electrodes for each one. The major ones are sodium (Na), potassium (K), and chloride (Cl). A major preanalytical error involves aggressive handling of the tube (shaking instead of gentle inversion) prior to analysis. It is frequently manifested by an artifactually high value for potassium. Ionized or free calcium, not bound to protein, can also be measured using an electrode specific for calcium.

Electrolyte measurements: Sodium (Na), Potassium (K), and Chloride (Cl)

To quantitate the major ions in patient plasma or serum using ion selective electrodes for each one

Expense: Low

Highly automated

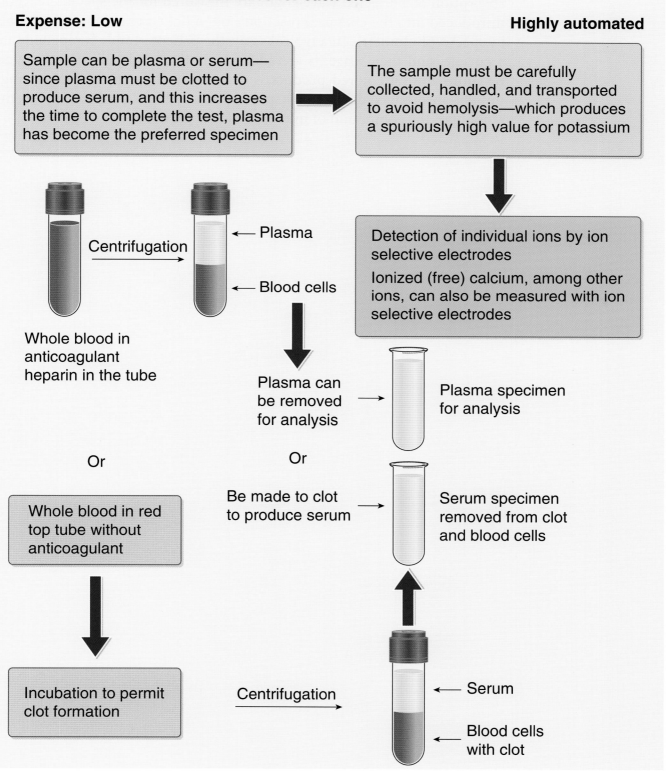

Sample can be plasma or serum—since plasma must be clotted to produce serum, and this increases the time to complete the test, plasma has become the preferred specimen

The sample must be carefully collected, handled, and transported to avoid hemolysis—which produces a spuriously high value for potassium

Plasma

Blood cells

Centrifugation

Whole blood in anticoagulant heparin in the tube

Detection of individual ions by ion selective electrodes

Ionized (free) calcium, among other ions, can also be measured with ion selective electrodes

Plasma can be removed for analysis

Plasma specimen for analysis

Or

Or

Whole blood in red top tube without anticoagulant

Be made to clot to produce serum

Serum specimen removed from clot and blood cells

Incubation to permit clot formation

Centrifugation

Serum

Blood cells with clot

ASSAYS MEASURING CONCENTRATION OF COMPOUNDS BY SPECTROPHOTOMETRY

There are many assays involving spectrophotometry as the detection method for quantitation of compounds in the clinical laboratory. Changes in light absorption at a selected wavelength are measured for the specific reagents introduced into the chemical reactions, often linked reactions, measurable by spectrophotometry. In a typical assay, the patient sample is pipetted into a cuvette, and then reagents are added to initiate and maintain chemical reactions until a colored product is generated. The extent of the change in light absorbance detected by spectrophotometry is proportional to the amount of the compound of interest which is present.

Assays measuring concentration of compounds or enzyme by spectrophotometry

To measure the concentration of a compound or the activity of a clinically relevant enzyme in patient plasma or serum by generating a compound in linked chemical reactions that can be measured spectrophotometrically

Expense: Low

Highly automated assays for most substances or activities measured

Sample is usually patient plasma or serum—for many assays, either can be used and for others, one or the other is specifically required

Common scenarios for testing and detection:

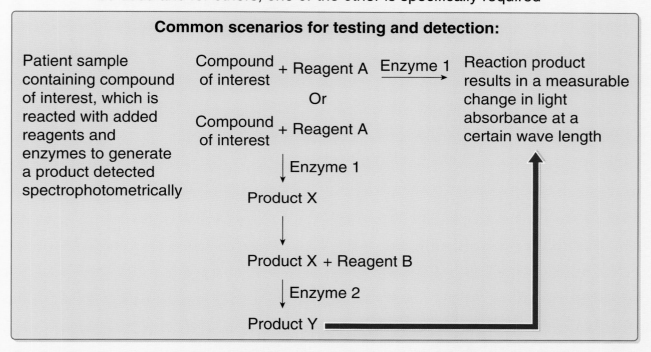

Patient sample containing compound of interest, which is reacted with added reagents and enzymes to generate a product detected spectrophotometrically

Compound of interest + Reagent A → Enzyme 1 →

Or

Compound of interest + Reagent A
↓ Enzyme 1
Product X
↓
Product X + Reagent B
↓ Enzyme 2
Product Y

Reaction product results in a measurable change in light absorbance at a certain wave length

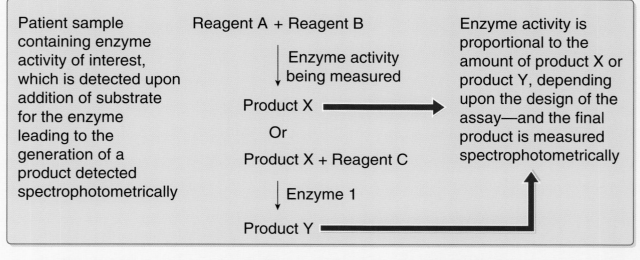

Patient sample containing enzyme activity of interest, which is detected upon addition of substrate for the enzyme leading to the generation of a product detected spectrophotometrically

Reagent A + Reagent B
↓ Enzyme activity being measured
Product X →

Or

Product X + Reagent C
↓ Enzyme 1
Product Y

Enzyme activity is proportional to the amount of product X or product Y, depending upon the design of the assay—and the final product is measured spectrophotometrically

Reagents A, B, and C, and enzymes 1 and 2 are all added to lead to the generation of a product that is proportional to the compound of interest or reflects the enzyme activity being measured

BLOOD GAS MEASUREMENTS

A whole blood specimen collected from an artery is injected into a blood gas analyzer which can determine pH, pO_2, and pCO_2. There are electrodes specific to hydrogen for pH, carbon dioxide for pCO_2, and oxygen for pO_2 in the blood gas instrument. These parameters are determined specifically for arterial blood, as the values in venous blood are markedly different.

Blood gas measurements

To quantitate the pH, pCO₂, and pO₂ in whole blood from a patient using ion selective electrodes for each one

Expense: Low

Requires injection of whole blood sample into instrument with no additional manipulation

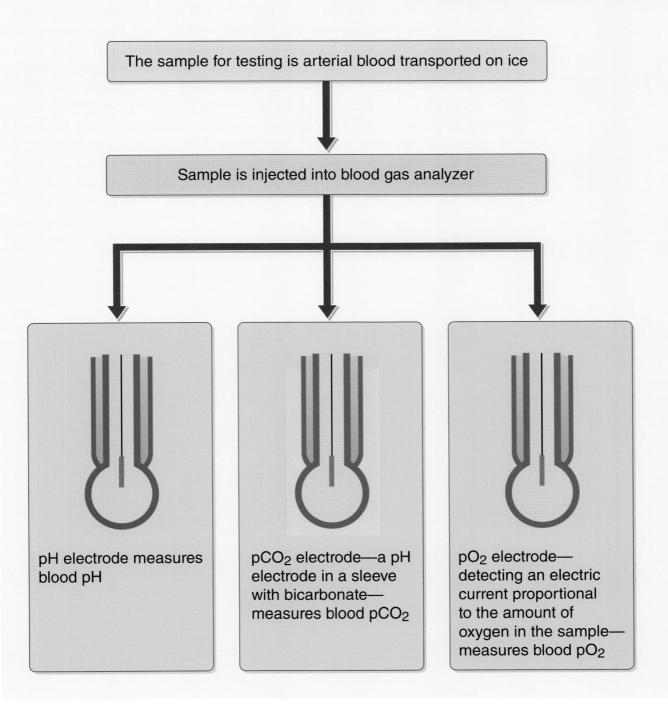

The sample for testing is arterial blood transported on ice

Sample is injected into blood gas analyzer

pH electrode measures blood pH

pCO₂ electrode—a pH electrode in a sleeve with bicarbonate—measures blood pCO₂

pO₂ electrode—detecting an electric current proportional to the amount of oxygen in the sample—measures blood pO₂

URINALYSIS

The first step in performing an analysis of urine is gross inspection of the urine for color and turbidity changes. A variety of colors other than yellow can be associated with a urine specimen, and samples from patients with a variety of conditions may be highly turbid. The chemical analysis of different compounds in the urine involves the use of a reagent pad that can detect many different compounds semiquantitatively. These include specific gravity, pH, leukocytes, nitrite, protein, glucose, ketones, urobilinogen, bilirubin, and blood. Some strips contain fewer pads than others. The strip is immersed in the urine for about one second, and the color changes of the reagent pads are noted at the appropriate time after removal of the strip from the urine. The semiquantitative measurement for each of the parameters can be read by spectrophotometry or viewed with the naked eye. In that circumstance, the results for each pad on the strip are established by comparison to pad colors associated with the different amounts of what is being measured. A sample of the urine can also be evaluated microscopically by placing a small volume of centrifuged urine on a glass slide. The urine sediment may reveal the presence of blood cells, epithelial cells, tumor cells, casts containing blood cells or other components, crystals, and other formed elements, including microorganisms.

Urinalysis

To measure selected constituents, including red and white blood cells in the urine by semiquantitative chemical reactions on a reagent strip; and to microscopically analyze the urine sediment after centrifugation for red and white blood cells, red and white blood cell casts, epithelial cells, and crystals of various types

Expense: Low

Can be completely manual or highly automated—sediment is examined microscopically which can be aided by automation in some instruments

There are two parts to a complete urinalysis

Chemical tests

Sediment analysis

Reagent pads on a dipstick change color at specified times when the compound of interest is present—after a brief dip of the stick into the urine

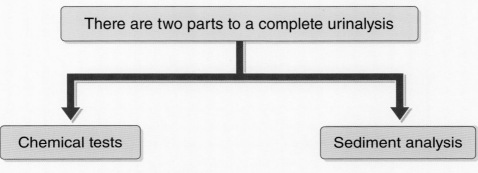

Urine is centrifuged and the concentrate is examined microscopically—notable findings include:
RBC
WBC
Collections of RBC or WBC in casts
A variety of cells from the urogenital tract
A variety of different crystals identifiable by size and shape

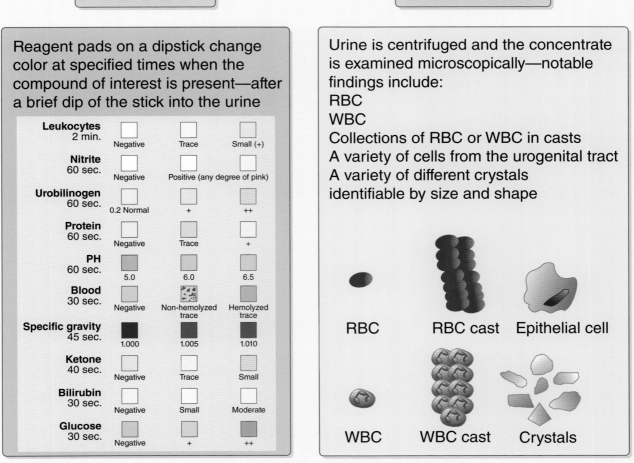

NEPHELOMETRY

In a nephelometry assay, a monoclonal antibody against an antigen of interest is added to a patient specimen, and then scattered or reflected light beamed into the test tube is measured. Antigen–antibody complexes scatter the light, and the amount of scattered light is proportional to the amount of antigen present in the patient sample. This method can detect and quantitate many compounds to which antibodies can become bound, including specific serum proteins such as immunoglobulins and complement proteins, as well as therapeutic drugs.

Nephelometry

To quantitate selected proteins and other compounds by measuring light scattering caused by antigen–antibody complexes

Expense: Moderate   **Semiautomated**

Sample of any body fluid is incubated with an antibody to the compound being measured

When the compound is present, antigen–antibody complexes form

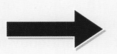

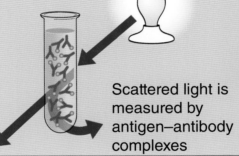

Antibody to the compound is the reagent added to the sample

Scattered light is measured by antigen–antibody complexes

Antigen is compound being measured

The amount of scattered light is proportional to the amount of compound being measured

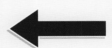

Antigen–antibody complexes scatter light from a beam of light shown through the sample

ENZYME-LINKED IMMUNOSORBENT ASSAY (ELISA)

The ELISA test can detect either antibodies or antigens in a patient's sample. For the test to detect antibodies, the antigen to which the antibody binds is fixed to the bottom of a small well of a tissue culture plate. The patient's serum is added to the small well, and if antibodies are present, they bind to the antigen. An antihuman antibody bound to an enzyme is then added. If the first antibody binds to the antigen fixed on the plate, that antibody from the patient will be detected by the second antibody to which the enzyme is linked. The substrate of the enzyme linked to the antibody is then added, and a colored product is generated. The amount of the antibody present is proportional to the amount of color change. To detect antigens, antibodies which bind the antigens of interest are fixed to the bottom of a dish. This allows for detection of a protein, hormone, drug, or other compound serving as the antigen in the test. After the antigen becomes bound to the antibody fixed onto the surface, a second antibody which is also specific for the ligand is then added. In this way, the ligand is the center of an antibody "sandwich." The second antibody added to the well has an enzyme linked to it. For detection, in the final step, the substrate of the enzyme which is bound to the antibody is added to the well. If the antigen of interest is present, a colored product will be generated which is proportional in intensity to the amount of antigen.

Enzyme-linked immunosorbent assay (ELISA)

To detect antibodies in patient plasma or serum by binding them to a corresponding antigen fixed to a surface; or to detect an antigen in patient plasma or serum by binding the antigen to corresponding antibodies fixed to a surface

Expense: Moderate

Semiautomated to almost fully automated

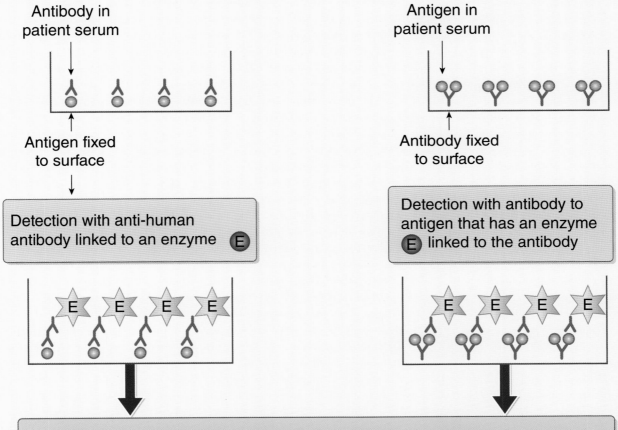

To detect antibodies in the patient's serum

To detect an antigen in the patient's serum

Antibodies are detected by binding to a corresponding antigen fixed to a surface

Antigens are detected by binding to corresponding antibodies fixed to a surface

Antibody in patient serum

Antigen in patient serum

Antigen fixed to surface

Antibody fixed to surface

Detection with anti-human antibody linked to an enzyme (E)

Detection with antibody to antigen that has an enzyme (E) linked to the antibody

Add uncolored substrate for enzyme and enzyme converts it to a colored product—the darker the color, the more antibody or antigen in the patient serum

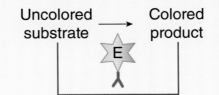

Uncolored substrate → Colored product

IMMUNOASSAY WITH ALL REAGENTS IN SOLUTION

An ELISA test can be performed completely in solution, without anything fixed to a surface, in a competitive binding assay. There is a linear relationship between the enzyme activity in this assay and the amount of antigen of interest in the patient's sample. The reagents are an antibody to an antigen of interest and the antigen of interest bound to an enzyme. When the antigen–enzyme complex is bound to antibody, there is no enzyme activity. If there is no antigen in the patient's sample, the antibody binds to the antigen–enzyme complex, and there is no enzyme activity. On the other hand, when antigen is present in the patient sample, free antigen is released from the antibody. The free antigen with attached enzyme becomes active, and the active enzyme converts an uncolored substrate to a colored product.

Fully automated immunoassay with all reagents in solution

To detect an antigen in any sample by using a competitive binding assay which has a linear increase in enzyme activity with increased antigen concentration

Expense: Low　　　　　　　　　　　　　　　　　　　　　**Automated**

No antigen in sample—negative test

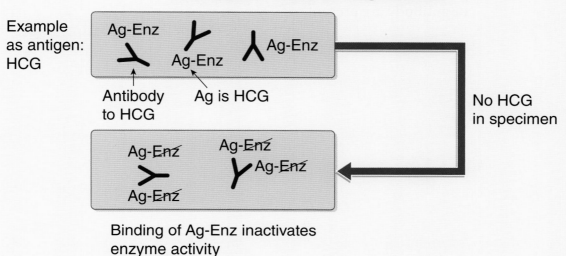

Example as antigen: HCG

Ag-Enz　Ag-Enz　Ag-Enz

Antibody to HCG　　Ag is HCG

No HCG in specimen

Ag-Enz　Ag-Enz　Ag-Enz　Ag-Enz

Binding of Ag-Enz inactivates enzyme activity
No signal

Antigen in sample—positive test

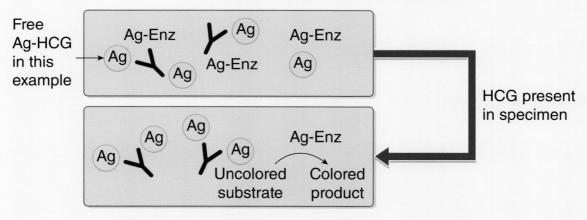

Free Ag-HCG in this example

Ag　Ag-Enz　Ag　Ag-Enz
Ag-Enz　Ag

HCG present in specimen

Ag　Ag　Ag-Enz
Ag　Ag
Uncolored substrate　Colored product

Free Ag-Enz allows enzyme to be active

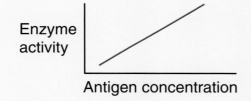

Enzyme activity

Antigen concentration

Enzyme conjugate activity is linearly proportional to antigen concentration in sample

Enz: Enzyme　　　　Ag: Antigen　　　　HCG: Human chorionic gonadotropin

LATEX AGGLUTINATION

In this simple manual test, a drop of latex particles, coated with either an antigen of interest or an antibody to a particular antigen, is mixed with the patient specimen. This test can detect antibodies in the specimen if the latex particles are bound with an antigen, or it can detect a specific antigen in the specimen if the latex particles are bound with antibodies to that antigen. The latter is depicted in the figure. The clumping of the latex particles is visible with the naked eye when adequate amounts of antigen or antibody are present.

Latex agglutination

To detect a compound in a liquid sample by allowing it to bind to latex particles with antibodies to the compound, which clumps the latex beads

Expense: Low   **Automated or manual**

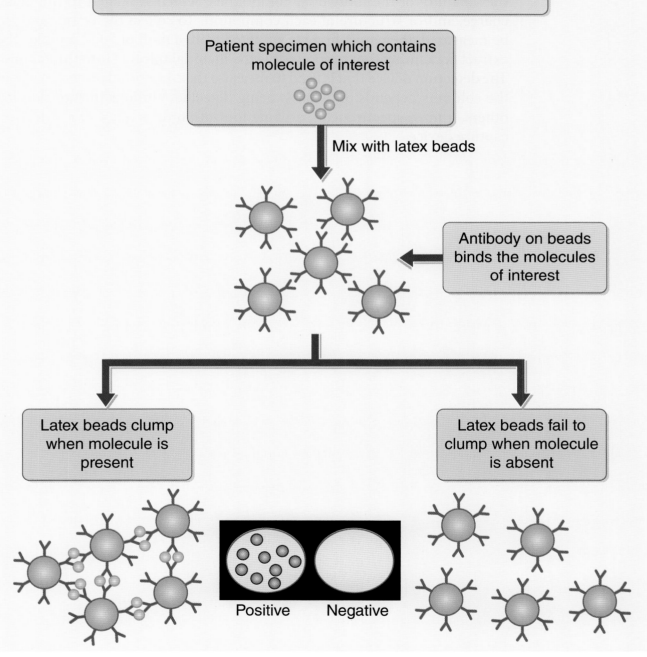

Goal of the test is to detect the presence of a compound in a patient specimen that visibly clumps latex particles

Patient specimen which contains molecule of interest

Mix with latex beads

Antibody on beads binds the molecules of interest

Latex beads clump when molecule is present

Latex beads fail to clump when molecule is absent

Positive   Negative

CHROMATOGRAPHY FOR SEPARATION, IDENTIFICATION, AND QUANTITATION OF SUBSTANCES IN BIOLOGIC FLUIDS

Chromatography involves the separation of compounds by a variety of different methods. The separation can be accomplished with different stable phases, to which compounds bind, and then are released from, and different mobile phases, which "push" the compounds through the stable phase. In gas chromatography, gas pushes solutes through a column to which volatile compounds attach and detach as the temperature within the system is increased. The separation of compounds within the column is based upon the volatility of the individual compounds, which is related to the mass, charge, and/or structure of each compound. To collect the compounds to be measured, they must first be extracted from a fluid or solid sample. The extract containing the compounds is the material injected into the column. The detection device that is used to measure the compounds emerging from the columns depends on what is being detected. Options include, among others, a mass spectrometer, a flame ionization detector, and an electron capture device.

Chromatography for separation, identification, and quantitation of substances in biologic fluids

To separate compounds in a single sample by one of several methods, so that individual compounds can be quantitated by an appropriate assay

Expense: High

Test requires manual processing and data analysis

Sample is extracted to remove extraneous molecules

Low-molecular-weight compounds

Large molecules such as proteins and nucleic acids

Analysis by gas chromatography (GC)

Analysis by high-performance liquid chromatography (HPLC)

Molecules in sample may require chemical derivatization to increase volatility in gas phase

Injection of samples into instrument with column separation

Column temperature increased to separate compounds

Mobile solvents and/or solvent pH altered to separate compounds

Signal

Time →

Compounds identified and quantitated using flame ionization (GC), spectroscopy (HPLC), mass spectrometry (GC and HPLC), or other detection method

MASS SPECTROMETRY FOR MOLECULAR IDENTIFICATION

Mass spectrometry is a method for molecular identification. In the mass spectrometer, individual compounds are fractured into smaller pieces. The pattern of the different pieces for an individual compound is highly specific. Information on the molecular weight of the compounds is also provided and is contributory to the identification of an individual molecule. Usually, mass spectrometry is preceded by some form of liquid chromatography, liquid–liquid, or gas chromatography to separate individual compounds from one another before they are identified. The pattern of molecular pieces of an individual molecule is known as its fingerprint. A mass spectrometer typically has a large database of fingerprints to which the fingerprint of an unknown molecule can be compared, thereby providing a percent likelihood for correct identification of a particular molecule.

Mass spectrometry for molecular identification

To identify a compound in a patient sample by causing it, by one of several techniques, to break into smaller ionized pieces; individual pieces are analyzed and detected by one of several technologies to create a pattern of the pieces that is characteristic for the compound; the pattern can be identified by comparison to fragment patterns from a large database of known compounds.

Expense: High

Semiautomated with high complexity of laboratory instrumentation

A patient sample is processed to render it suitable for analysis

Molecular compounds of interest are isolated from other molecules in sample, commonly by liquid chromatography or gas chromatography

In tandem mass spectrometry there are multiple rounds of mass spectrometry. Molecules are ionized and then separated by mass-to-charge ratio (m/z). Ions of a particular m/z ratio are then selected and split into smaller fragment ions which are separated by m/z ratio, detected, and quantitated

In the mass spectrometer, individual molecules are broken into different size mass fragments and ionized, creating a "fingerprint" for each individual molecule

The fingerprint of the molecule in the patient specimen is compared to a large library of molecular fingerprints

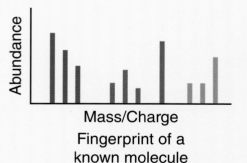

Fingerprint of a known molecule

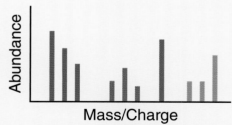

Fingerprint of compound in patient specimen

Molecule is identified because fingerprints match with very high percentage of agreement

NEWBORN SCREENING BY LIQUID CHROMATOGRAPHY/ MASS SPECTROMETRY (LC-MS)

Newborn screening tests and the methodologies used for the tests vary from one jurisdiction to another. In general, after 24 hours of life, whole blood is obtained from the puncture of the heel of a neonate. The blood is placed onto the card in multiple drops, with each one intended for a different screening test. The compounds to be measured that are related to the diseases for which the newborn is being screened are extracted from the blood spot on the paper, and then isolated by liquid chromatography in the method depicted. A mass spectrometer can be used to identify and quantitate the compounds of interest. For blood samples containing compounds in abnormal concentrations, a positive newborn screening test is generated. This leads to further evaluation to determine if the disease suggested by the screening test result is present.

Newborn screening by liquid chromatography/mass spectrometry (LC-MS)

To detect and measure substances in newborn blood which are suggestive of certain diseases using liquid chromatography combined with mass spectrometry

Expense: High for instrumentation; moderate for test performance

Semiautomated with high-complexity instrumentation

After 24 h of life, heel of neonate is punctured to obtain whole blood—which is spotted onto a special card and sent to a central laboratory

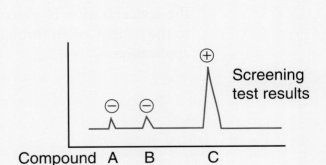

Blood spots on card

Molecular compounds of interest are extracted from a portion of the blood spot and separated by liquid chromatography

Portion of 1 blood spot

LC-MS analysis

A tandem mass spectrometer identifies the compounds of interest and quantifies the amount of each—and those compounds in higher concentrations than the reference range are "positive" in the newborn screening test

Screening test results

Compound   A   B   C

Confirmation of positive test for compound C is performed to determine if result is true-positive

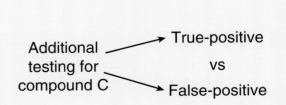

Additional testing for compound C

True-positive

vs

False-positive

7 Point-of-Care Testing Methods

POINT-OF-CARE GLUCOSE TESTING

Using a small device which is handheld or attached to the body of a patient undergoing glucose monitoring on a regular basis, a blood sample is obtained. The glucose concentration in the plasma of the patient mixes with reagents within the device and generates a signal proportional to the concentration of glucose in the sample. The result is then displayed to the patient, often through a window in the device or through a mobile application.

Point-of-care glucose testing

To quantitate glucose in blood using a small handheld device

Expense: Low

After sample is added to test strip, testing is automated

Result display

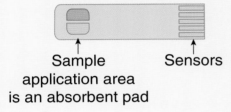

Test strip with sample   Glucometer

Top-down view of strip

Sample application area is an absorbent pad   Sensors

Side view of strip

RBC, WBC, and platelets stay on top of absorbent pad

Plasma passes through absorbent pad

Top-down view of strip below absorbent pad

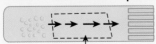

Reagents that react with glucose embedded here as plasma moves toward sensors

A blood sample, which is commonly from a finger stick, is applied to a test strip

Sample application occurs onto an absorbent pad that separates blood cells from plasma

Glucose within plasma mixes with reagents embedded on test strip as plasma moves toward sensors

Enzyme reactions with glucose as substrate produce electrons detected by sensors at the end of the test strip inserted into glucometer

Sensor signal is proportional to concentration of glucose in sample, which is shown in the result display window of the glucometer

POINT-OF-CARE IMMUNOASSAY ON TEST STRIP

Test strips which identify the presence of a specific compound in a liquid sample have antibodies to the compound fixed at a certain location on the strip. When the sample is applied, fluid migration occurs with a wicking action out of the sample application spot. As the sample with the compound of interest that can bind to the fixed antibody moves along the strip, it is captured by the antibody, creating a band visible to the naked eye. For all assays involving test strips, there is also a control band which must appear to indicate that the assay is valid. If the control band is not visible, the test result is uninterpretable because it indicates a failure of the assay.

Point-of-care immunoassay on a test strip

To identify the presence of a compound in a liquid sample using test strips with antibodies to the compound fixed to the strip; designed for point-of-care use

Cost: Moderate

Manual test requiring interpretation

Negative test

Top-down view of strip

Side view of test strip: Before application of sample

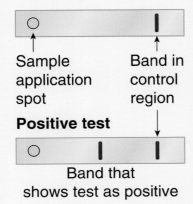

Sample application spot

Band in control region

Positive test

Band that shows test as positive

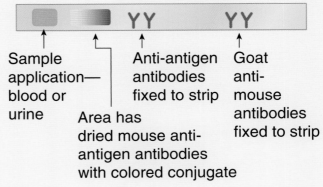

Sample application—blood or urine

Area has dried mouse anti-antigen antibodies with colored conjugate

Anti-antigen antibodies fixed to strip

Goat anti-mouse antibodies fixed to strip

Negative test
Fluid migration with wicking action out of sample application spot

Side view of test strip after sample application—antigen (Ag) is absent

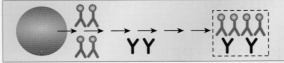

Sample added to well

Solubilizes mouse anti-antigen antibodies with colored conjugate

No antigen in sample

Goat anti-mouse antibodies bind mouse anti-antigen antibodies to make 1 band in control region

Positive test
Example antigen is HCG—in a pregnancy test

Side view of test strip—antigen (Ag) is present

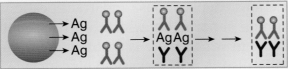

Ag: Antigen

Mouse anti-antigen antibodies fixed to strip bind Ag—and the solubilized mouse anti-antigen antibodies with the colored conjugate also bind Ag to form a colored band where fixed antibodies are imbedded onto strip

Goat anti-mouse antibodies fixed to strip bind excess solubilized mouse anti-antigen antibodies to create a second colored band—bands shown within dashed lines

8 Methods Involving Chromosomal Analysis and Molecular Genetics

Chromosomal Analysis

THE KARYOTYPE

A karyotype analysis involves the use of fresh viable tissue cells grown in culture and arrested in the stage of cell division known as metaphase. In metaphase, the chromosomes condense and become distinguishable from the other chromosomes, as they align in the center of the dividing cell. The process of karyotyping involves the pairing and ordering of all the chromosomes, providing a genome-wide view of the individual's chromosomes. The karyotype can reveal missing chromosomes, extra chromosomes, or deletions, duplications, and translocations of parts of chromosomes. A common abnormality which can be identified by karyotyping is Down syndrome in which there is trisomy of chromosome 21. Other commonly identified disorders using karyotyping include Turner syndrome, Klinefelter syndrome, and fragile X syndrome.

The Karyotype

To evaluate chromosomal structure and number, and banding pattern

Cost: Expensive

Manual test with detailed interpretation

Human somatic cells have 46 chromosomes with 22 homologous autosomal pairs and 2 sex chromosomes—XX in females and XY in males

Blood sample collected in heparin-containing vacuum tube

→

Portion of sample placed into tissue culture medium with mitogens to promote lymphocyte proliferation or without mitogens

→

After 16–72 h of incubation time, colcemid added to arrest cell division and ethidium bromide added to elongate chromosomes

Slides are stained with Giemsa stain to produce characteristic dark and light bands

←

Nuclei are dropped onto slide to optimize spreading of metaphase chromosomes

←

Cells are ruptured while nuclei remain intact

Microscope or imaging software used to capture metaphase cells and enable karyotyping

→

Evaluation for numerical abnormalities and structural rearrangements by counting chromosomes and assessing the banding pattern for each chromosome

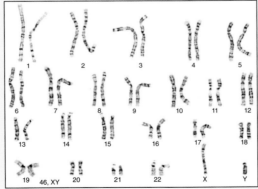

A normal male karyotype
(Courtesy of Dr Ferrin Wheeler)

Description of karyotype is total number of chromosomes, the sex chromosomes, description of any abnormality
Example: 47, XY, +21 is a male with trisomy 21.

FLUORESCENCE *IN SITU* HYBRIDIZATION (FISH)

Fluorescence *in situ* Hybridization (FISH) is a well-established technique for the detection of numerous structural genome abnormalities. These include deletions, insertions, and translocations associated with genomic material which is missing, redundantly copied, or moved to other locations within the genome. As such, this is a common technique used in cancer diagnosis because many cancers have well-known genome alterations. The figure depicts translocation of genes in a sample of cancer cells.

FISH proceeds by first creating a collection of short DNA sequences representing a target of interest, such as a gene which is commonly translocated in a specific cancer. These short sequences are called "probes," and they are modified through the addition of a fluorescent label to each fragment. The principle of this test is that the fluorescently labeled probes will bind specifically to a region in the sample DNA to which they are complementary, and the presence of the associated fluorescent tag will indicate the presence, abundance, and chromosomal location of the target sequence.

Fluorescence *in situ* hybridization (FISH)

To detect the chromosomal location of specific genes using fluorescent single-stranded DNA probes which bind to complementary sequences of denatured, single-stranded patient DNA in metaphase chromosomes, viewed by fluorescence microscopy

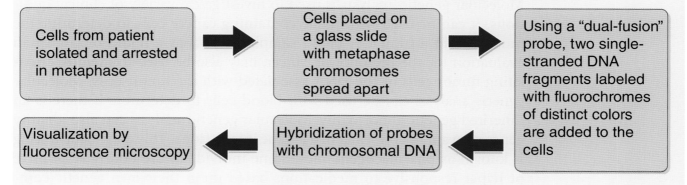

Example of results using a
green (G) and a red (R) probe

NORMAL

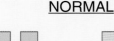

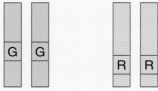

Two different homologous
chromosomes—one
labeled by green DNA
probe and one by red
DNA probe

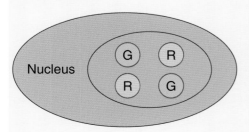

Genes located by probes
and fluorescence microscopy of
chromosomes show no
translocation of genes probed

ABNORMAL

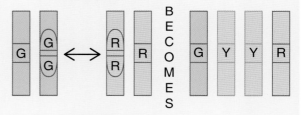

Neoplastic cell with
reciprocal translocation
shows split signals for
both green and red probes
    When chromosome
fragments are exchanged,
two yellow (red + green) (Y)
signals are generated

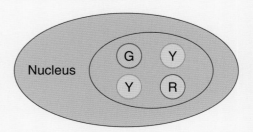

Two normal chromosomes
and two "derivative"
chromosomes identified
by fluorescence microscopy

Molecular Genetic Testing

CLINICAL TESTING USING MOLECULAR GENETIC ANALYSIS

Molecular genetic analysis is used to investigate a variety of clinical questions. It can be used with tissue containing cancer cells to determine the mutations in a tumor. A blood sample, known as a liquid biopsy in an evaluation for the presence of cancer, may also be used to identify circulating tumor cells or the DNA associated with the tumor cells. Molecular genetic analysis can be used with blood cells to determine if there is an inherited genetic abnormality. Molecular genetic analysis can also identify genes relevant to abnormal drug–gene interactions. This diagnostic testing is known as pharmacogenomics. Some individuals are poorly responsive or hyper-responsive to medications based upon their own genetic composition. Finally, a sample which may contain infectious organisms can be studied with molecular genetics to assess for the presence and definitive identification of organisms.

Clinical testing using molecular genetic analysis: An overview

To detect genetic variations/mutations in tumors, to establish malignant and non-malignant diagnoses, to identify adverse drug–gene interactions, and to find infectious organisms

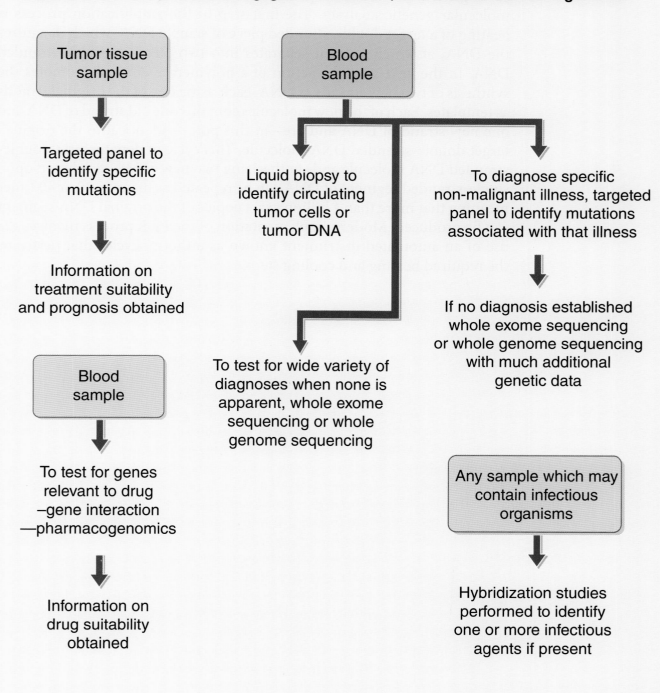

Molecular Genetic Testing: PCR Methods

POLYMERASE CHAIN REACTION (PCR)

Polymerase chain reaction is a methodology that allows for the amplification of small segments of DNA. This amplification of the DNA is critical to generate an adequate quantity of material to perform many different molecular genetic analyses. The first step in the amplification process is heating of a target double-stranded piece of sample DNA, which denatures the DNA, at which point it separates into two pieces of single-stranded DNA. In the next step, the action of a polymerase enzyme promotes the synthesis of two new strands of DNA, each using one of the original strands as templates. Each of the new molecules contains one old strand of DNA and one new strand of DNA and are—at this point—identical to the original, target double-stranded DNA molecule. This cycle of denaturing a double-stranded DNA molecule and synthesizing two new copies each based upon single-stranded segment of DNA can be repeated as many as 30 or 40 times meaning that more than 1 billion exact copies of the original DNA segment can be produced. Modern implementation of the PCR process involves the use of an automated instrument known as a thermocycler that performs the required heating and cooling steps.

Polymerase chain reaction (PCR)

PCR specimen: DNA extracted from blood, body fluid, disrupted tissue, or environmental source

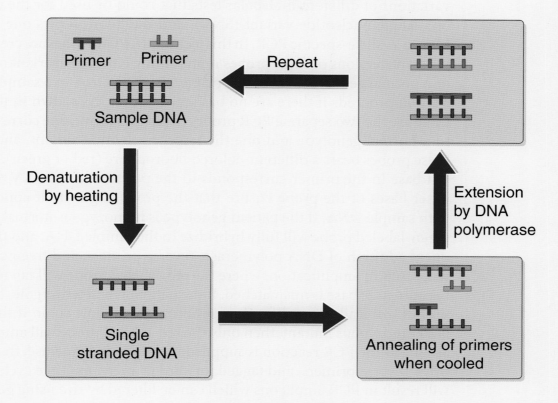

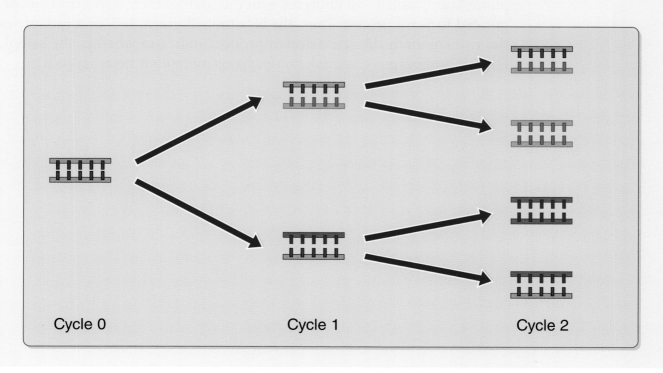

DETECTION OF A GENOMIC ALTERATION USING PCR

Having discussed the principle of PCR, this figure illustrates how PCR can be used to identify a genomic alteration in a patient sample. The example used here is for a patient with a single point mutation. There are many variations of different molecular tests that could be used for the detection of a single nucleotide variant (SNV), and the figure shows one such test known as allele-specific PCR. In this technique, PCR probes are created with different versions of these probes representing either the variant of interest or a normal genotype. When the primers bind to DNA in a sample, amplification proceeds if there are no base mismatches. As shown in the figure, there are the two separate PCR probes described above, one corresponding to a normal genotype and one the target nucleotide variant, and each of these probes bears a different-colored fluorophore (red or green). The very last base in the primer corresponds to the position of the SNV, while the other bases of the probe ensure that the probe aligns itself appropriately with sample DNA. If the patient genotype is homozygous normal, then the green-labeled probe will fully hybridize to the sample DNA, and the subsequent addition of DNA polymerase, reverse primers, and free nucleotides will result in amplification, where the red-labeled probe will fail to amplify because its 3′ base is mismatched. If the patient is a heterozygote, then both probes will lead to amplification, resulting in a yellow color. If the patient is a homozygous mutant, then only the red-labeled probe will amplify. And as long as the PCR reaction is supplied with DNA polymerase, free nucleotides, reverse primers, and tagged forward primers, multiple cycles of PCR will result in PCR amplicons which can be filtered by size using gel electrophoresis and which will fluoresce with the color of their respectively incorporated forward primer. Thus, the bias toward green, red, or a mixture of the two colors in the size-selected product indicates whether the sample DNA is homozygous normal, homozygous mutant, or heterozygous.

Detection of a genomic alteration using PCR

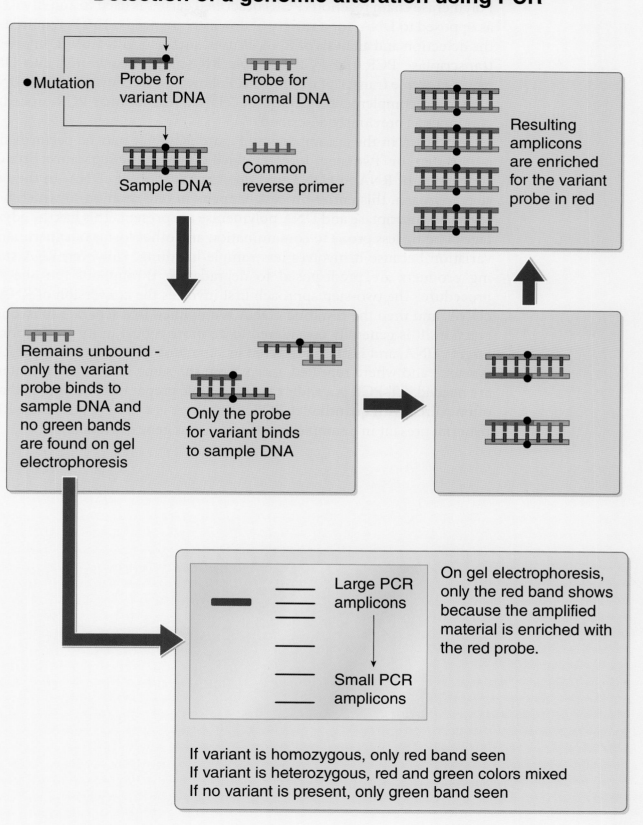

REVERSE TRANSCRIPTION PCR

Polymerase chain reaction (PCR) described earlier is used to amplify RNA, as opposed to DNA, for a variety of downstream needs. This is required for the detection and analysis of RNA viruses, such as SARS-CoV-2. In reverse transcriptase PCR (RT-PCR), sample RNA is first converted into DNA using a reverse transcriptase enzyme. Following this conversion into DNA, known as "complementary DNA" or "cDNA," the familiar PCR procedure continues as previously described.

As shown in the accompanying Figure, RT-PCR may be performed in a "one-step" or "two-step" format, which differs in the separation between conversion of RNA to cDNA and the amplification of cDNA. In the one-step approach, this entire process happens in one reaction in which both reverse transcriptase and DNA polymerase are present. This has the advantage of being less prone to contamination and other forms of experimental variation because it involves less sample handling. However, RNA starting products are predisposed to degradation throughout the one-step procedure. The two-step approach first involves the conversion of RNA to cDNA, and then the resulting cDNA is amplified in a separate subsequent reaction. It is generally considered to be more robust in its production of target cDNA, and is often preferred in situations where input sample RNA is scarce and where repeated assays from the same sample input material are needed. RT-PCR is a widely useful sample preparation technique that is often paired with quantitative PCR when there is a need to quantitate RNA material present in a sample in order to assess gene expression.

Reverse transcription PCR

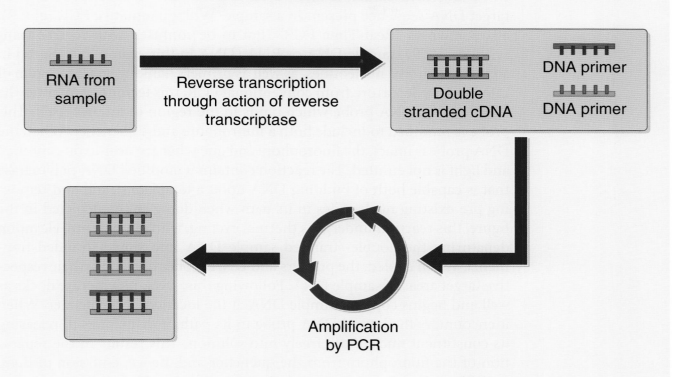

One-step method

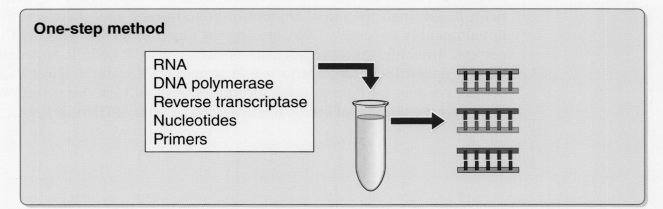

Two-step method

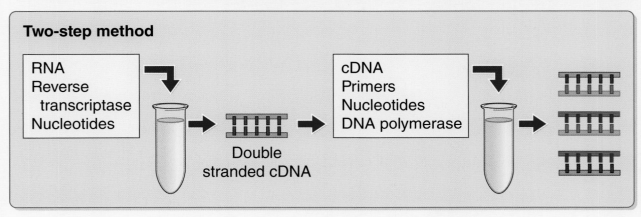

QUANTITATIVE PCR

PCR, described earlier, is often used to detect the abundance of a given target DNA sequence present in a sample. With quantitative PCR (qPCR), also known as "Real-Time PCR" (not to be confused with reverse transcription PCR), sample DNA or RNA (DNA in this example) is placed in solution with free nucleotides, as well as primers flanking a target region of interest. In a departure from conventional PCR, this technique involves the addition of a DNA probe which binds to the region of interest itself. This probe is modified to include both a fluorophore and a quencher. When the DNA probe is intact, the fluorophore and quencher are near to one another, and light is not emitted. The reaction contains a modified DNA polymerase that is capable both of building DNA upon a template strand and removing pre-existing nucleotides in its path when doing so. As depicted in the figure, this reaction undergoes thermal cycling, with temperature elevation denaturing the double-stranded sample DNA into single-stranded fragments. When cooled, the primers and DNA probes dock onto their respective target areas of sample DNA. Following this, DNA polymerase docks as well and begins copying sample DNA at the location of the primer. When it encounters the bound DNA probe in its path, it dismantles it, releasing its constituent nucleotides freely into solution. This results in the separation of the fluorophore from the quencher and, hence, emission of light. As PCR cycles repeat, the abundance of accumulated light scales exponentially, based upon the initial amount of bound probe and, therefore, the initial quantity of sample DNA bearing the target sequence. This light is detected over time and the intensity of light per PCR cycle is recorded. Greater quantities of target sequence in sample DNA result in fewer PCR cycles necessary for light to reach a certain threshold value for detection. The lower the number of cycles, the larger the amount of DNA or RNA.

Quantitative PCR

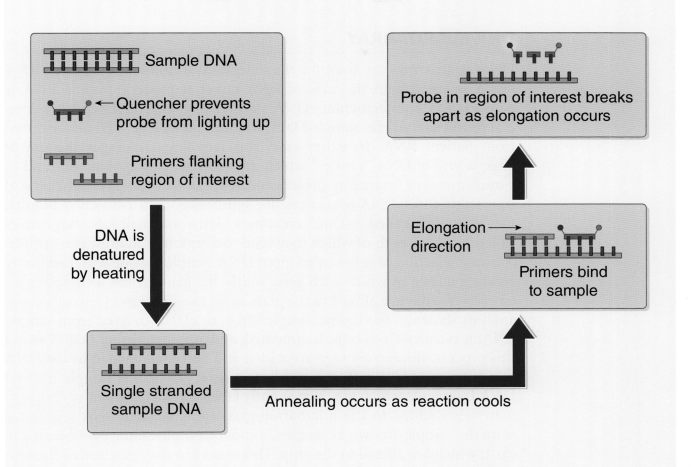

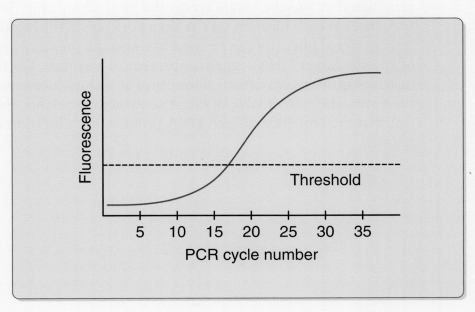

Molecular Genetic Testing: Array/Hybridization Methods

DNA MICROARRAY

DNA microarrays are used for the detection of numerous DNA or RNA target sequences. In the case of RNA target sequences, sample RNA is converted to "complementary DNA" or "cDNA" as an initial step. Therefore, this procedure utilizes sample DNA, whether patient-derived or converted from patient RNA. In either case, this technique leverages the use of large arrays of DNA "probes" which are short sequences that will bind to complementary fragments present in the input sample. Typically, tens of thousands short DNA sequences are synthesized and covalently bonded to a glass slide called a "chip," creating a "lawn" of small DNA sequences called "probes," each of which may bind to a region of interest in a sample. A broad selection of genes in an input DNA sample may be searched for by creating a lawn in which each gene within the genome has a complementary short sequence affixed to the glass slide. In a common form of sample analysis shown in the figure, sample DNA, or cDNA derived from sample RNA, is purified from cells, fragmented, and amplified using PCR. During this process, fluorescent tags are added and become attached to the DNA copies generated by PCR. This results in a library of smaller sample-derived DNA fragments which are fluorescently labeled. When patient or "library" material is added to the microarray glass slide, labeled DNA sequences from the sample, known as "targets," bind to complementary probes, if any exist, which are affixed to the chip. This results in the detection of fluorescent signal at specific locations on the microarray chip. Since the probe sequences at each location on the lawn are known, the locations with fluorescent signal intensity can be used to assess the presence and the quantity of specific target DNA sequences present in a sample. On the microarray instrument, a camera detects florescence at various locations, and converts the florescence into a table of target sequence abundances based upon the fact that the sequence of each DNA probe at each location on this chip is known.

DNA microarray

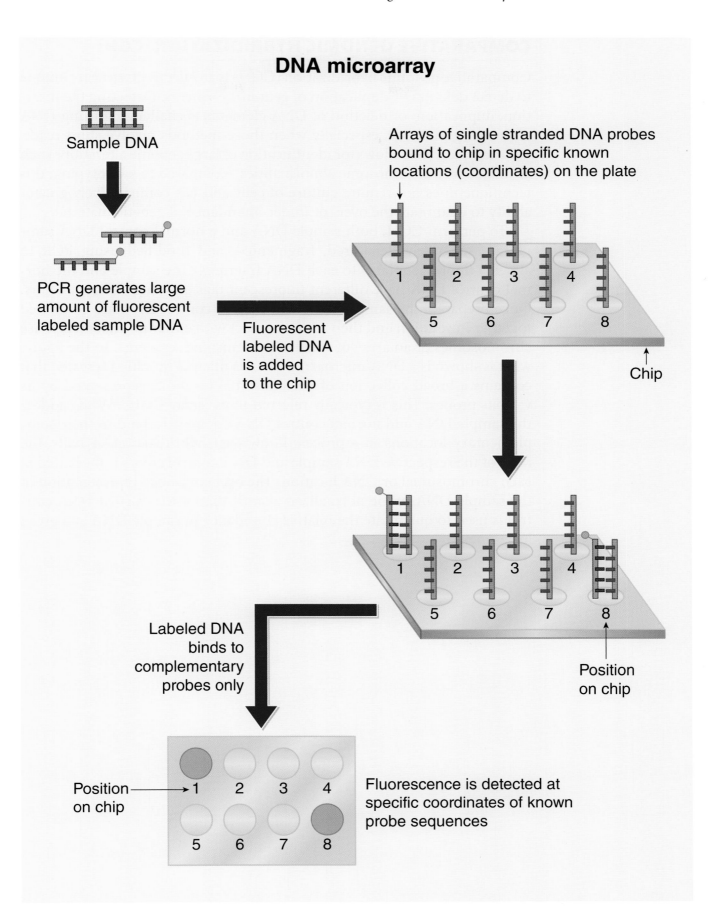

Sample DNA

PCR generates large amount of fluorescent labeled sample DNA

Fluorescent labeled DNA is added to the chip

Arrays of single stranded DNA probes bound to chip in specific known locations (coordinates) on the plate

Chip

Labeled DNA binds to complementary probes only

Position on chip

Position on chip

Fluorescence is detected at specific coordinates of known probe sequences

COMPARATIVE GENOMIC HYBRIDIZATION (CGH)

Comparative genomic hybridization (CGH) is an effective testing technique to detect deletion or duplication of genomic elements. Detecting the insertion, duplication, or deletion of DNA elements is challenging using DNA sequencing methods, especially when those methods involve short reads. For example, CGH allows for identification of large genome alterations such as unbalanced chromosome abnormalities. Compared to karyotyping, this technique does not require culture of cells and has comparatively greater ability to quantitate the over- or under-abundance of genetic material.

To perform CGH, both sample DNA and a normal control DNA sample are separately denatured, fragmented, and modified using PCR to attach a fluorescent label to each DNA fragment. The sample and the normal control DNA have different fluorescent tags emitting different colors. Once prepared, the sample DNA and normal control DNA are combined together in solution and then added to react with either normal metaphase chromosomes or an array of smaller chromosome segments. In the figure, what is shown is a DNA microarray where a microarray chip is created that contains a broad collection of chromosomal locations represented by its various probes. This is typically referred to as "array CGH." When added, the sample DNA and normal control DNA compete to bind to their complementary locations in a process known as "hybridization." Finally, the ratio of the respective DNA sample and DNA control colors is measured at each chromosomal or DNA location. The over- or under-representation of the sample DNA probe normalized against that of the normal DNA control is used to quantitate the relative abundance of sample DNA at a given location.

Comparative genomic hybridization (CGH)

Sample DNA   Normal DNA

DNA denaturation, fragmentation, and fluorescent label attached to each fragment

• Fluorescent tag for DNA from patient sample

• Fluorescent tag for DNA from normal control sample

1 2 3
4 5 6 7
8 9 10

DNA is added onto an array of chromosome segments

1 2 3
4 5 6 7
8 9 10

Both sample and normal DNA bind to complementary chromosome regions

Binding of:

Sample DNA   Both   Normal DNA

1 2 3
4 5 6 7
8 9 10

Relative abundance between sample and normal DNA is read as fluorescent color in chromosomal regions

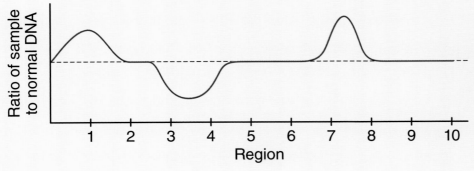

Relative abundance is plotted as the ratio of sample to normal DNA for each region

DETECTION OF A GENOMIC ALTERATION USING CGH

This figure shows how CGH can be used to identify a genomic alteration in a patient sample. The example shown is from a patient with a partial deletion of a chromosome who carries a diagnosis of Cri du Chat syndrome with a partial deletion of the short arm of chromosome 5. The principle of the test requires separately fragmenting normal DNA and patient (sample) DNA, and comparing results using each set of fragments. Separately colored fluorescent tags are added, and these tagged DNA fragments compete for binding to a collection of chromosomes in a metaphase spread.

In the figure, normal DNA labeled with a green fluorophore and sample DNA labeled with a red fluorophore have been fragmented, and each of these is added to the collection of chromosomes in a metaphase spread. If both the normal and sample DNA contain equal amounts of a specific chromosomal region, then their fragments will bind in equal amounts to that corresponding section of the metaphase chromosomes. The combination of the two fluorophores will result in a yellow color. Conversely, if the sample DNA is missing a chromosomal region, such as having a deletion in the short arm of chromosome 5, then only the normal DNA will bind to that chromosomal region, resulting in that region appearing green.

For higher resolution, the balance of fluorescence from red to yellow to green can be quantitated using a fluorescence detector and whole metaphase chromosomes may be replaced with arrays of specific chromosomal segments spread over a plate. This method, commonly referred to as array CGH, is depicted in the previous figure.

Detection of a genetic alteration using comparative genomic hybridization (CGH)

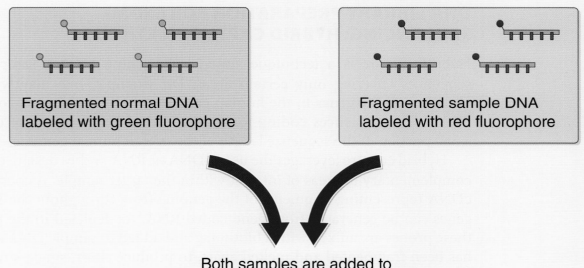

Fragmented normal DNA labeled with green fluorophore

Fragmented sample DNA labeled with red fluorophore

Both samples are added to metaphase chromosomes in a spread

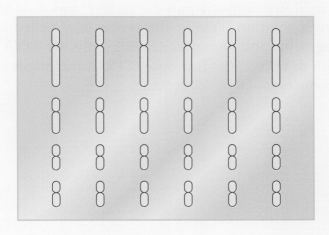

Metaphase chromosomes are arranged on a surface

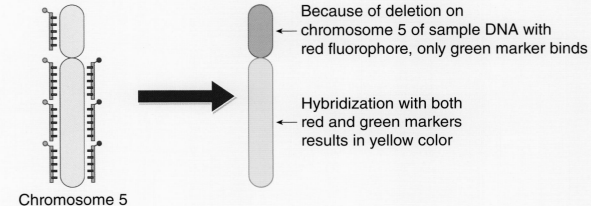

Chromosome 5

Because of deletion on chromosome 5 of sample DNA with red fluorophore, only green marker binds

Hybridization with both red and green markers results in yellow color

Molecular Genetic Testing: Nucleic Acid Sequencing Methods

DNA LIBRARY PREPARATION FOR EXOME SEQUENCING: HYBRID CAPTURE METHODS

Hybrid capture is a technique aimed at enriching a DNA sample for sequences covering only certain areas. For example, one may wish to sequence all the genes in the human genome, of which there are roughly 30,000. The sequences coding for the individual genes represent only a small portion of the sequence length of the overall human genome.

Hybrid capture leverages the use of DNA or RNA probes designed to be complementary to areas of interest within the target sample. A cocktail of cDNA representing fragments of the genome from throughout the 30,000 genes can be generated from gene-coded RNA. As depicted in the figure, these probes are affixed with a biotin tag and added to sample DNA after it has been fragmented and melted apart, to produce short, single-stranded DNA fragments. In solution, these probes bind only to DNA fragments containing complementary sequences. The biotin attached to the probes is used to selectively pull the probes, and their attached DNA fragments, out of solution. Finally, the probes are melted off of their sample DNA fragments and removed, leaving only the DNA fragments enriched for regions of interest. This pool of DNA fragments can then be processed for downstream DNA sequencing.

Library preparation for exome sequencing: hybrid capture method

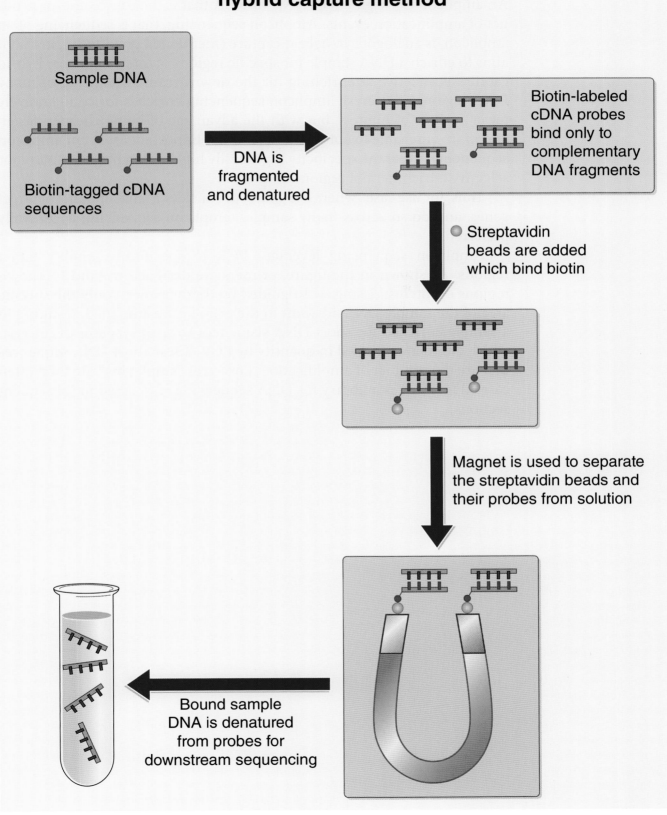

DNA LIBRARY PREPARATION FOR TARGETED SEQUENCING: AMPLICON GENERATION METHOD

An amplicon is a segment of DNA or RNA that is the source and/or product of amplification events. Amplicon sequencing, that is sequencing of an amplicon, is analogous to hybrid capture (mentioned previously), in that it aims to enrich a DNA sample for specific regions of interest. Where hybrid capture is effective at enriching for the downstream sequencing of many DNA regions of interest, amplicon sequencing enriches for comparatively fewer regions of interest, but with the advantage of being cheaper, faster, and more amenable to automation. Another important aspect of amplicon sequencing is that the specificity is generally higher than hybrid capture for selective enrichment of regions of interest.

Thus, for use cases where the goal is to consider a smaller panel of target genes, and do so across many samples, amplicon sequencing is generally preferred.

Amplicon sequencing leverages PCR to specifically amplify target regions. As shown in the figure, primers are designed to bind to known regions of interest. Using PCR, guided by these primers, only the specific area of the sample DNA adjacent to the primers are amplified, resulting in a sample enriched for short DNA sequences covering regions of interest, which are then increased in quantity by PCR. These short DNA sequences that are the product of amplification, known as "amplicons," are then often carried forward as a library for DNA sequencing (discussed in subsequent sections).

Library preparation for targeted sequencing: amplicon generation method

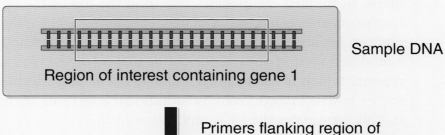

Sample DNA

Region of interest containing gene 1

Primers flanking region of interest are used to amplify these segments by PCR

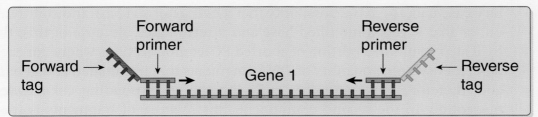

Forward primer

Reverse primer

Forward → tag

← Reverse tag

Gene 1

Multiple PCR cycles amplify multiple genes of interest; only gene 1 is shown

Short "tag" sequences of nucleotides (red and orange here) identify the sequence as derived from the specific amplicon for the region containing gene 1

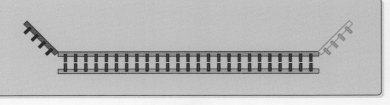

This amplicon, one of many, is the material used for downstream sequencing

Sequencing of the region of interest establishes the sequence of gene 1

SANGER SEQUENCING

In its contemporary form, this method is properly known as "Sanger Sequencing by Capillary Electrophoresis" with two methodologic components. In the first component, shown in the top of the figure, input DNA fragments are placed into a matrix containing DNA polymerase and free nucleotides, and are allowed to replicate by PCR. This reaction also contains a modified version of each nucleotide that is labeled with an excitable fluorophore which is color-coded and also chemically modified so that when such a base is incorporated, no additional bases can be incorporated after it. This terminates the PCR replication of the DNA fragment at the point at which this nucleotide is incorporated. In this reaction, there are both normal base pairs and a smaller proportion of modified base pairs, such that, for example, there is both a normal guanine and a modified guanine. As a result, at each base position where PCR attempts to add a complementary base pair, there is a possibility that it gets a normal base and continues on, or that it gets a modified base and it terminates. Because of this, the PCR step results in a portion of aborted PCR amplifications where, for each base, there is some quantity of DNA fragments that terminated at that base and, therefore, fragments that end with the corresponding color-coded nucleotide. In the second component, this mixture of fragments is then injected into a gel-filled capillary system where they separate by size, with smaller fragments moving faster than larger ones. This is precise enough to spatially separate fragments that differ by as little as one base in size. A laser is located at the end of the capillary to excite the fluorophores, and each fragment emits the wavelength associated with its respective terminating nucleotide label. This results in a series of colors ordered by size and, since size order represents base order, this color series can be read out as a sequence of bases known as an "electropherogram."

Sanger sequencing

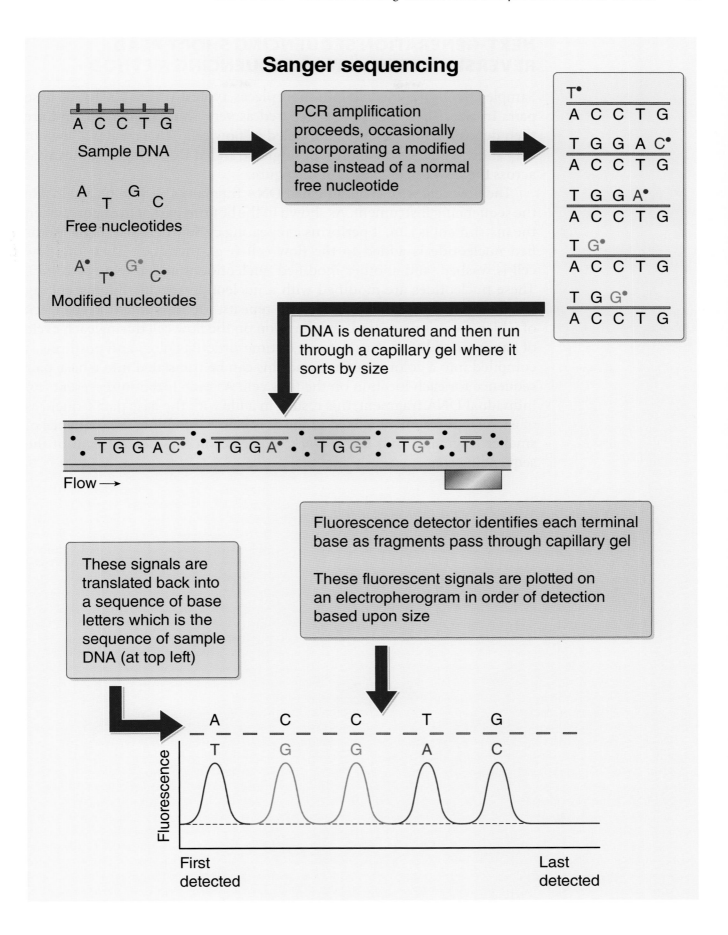

NEXT-GENERATION SEQUENCING SHORT READ: REVERSIBLE TERMINATOR SEQUENCING METHOD

Sample DNA is fragmented into short pieces, typically from 300 to 500 base pairs in size. These pieces are prepared as very short sequences, and are then deposited onto a glass slide called a "flow cell." This creates a lawn of very short sequences in a forest of single-stranded DNA fragments arrayed across the flow cell as shown in the figure.

The flow cell, with all its attached DNA fragments, is then placed inside the sequencing instrument. As shown in the bottom part of the figure, when the instrument is run, it performs a repeating cycle wherein a single modified nucleotide is added to the flow cell (e.g., thymine). Then the flow cell is washed, and another modified nucleotide is added (e.g., cytosine). These nucleotides are modified with a nucleotide-specific fluorescent tag (i.e., color-coded). Thus, as this cycle repeats, the instrument keeps track of which color is present in each location on the flow cell during each cycle of base pair addition. This data set of time-ordered colors and positions is compiled into a color sequence, and this can be translated into a base pair sequence for each location on the flow cell. As each location represents an individual DNA fragment, this results in a file with the base pair sequences of each DNA fragment affixed to the flow cell. Assembling the sequence of smaller fragments into larger DNA sequences occurs downstream of the sequencing step.

Next generation sequencing, short read: reversible terminator method

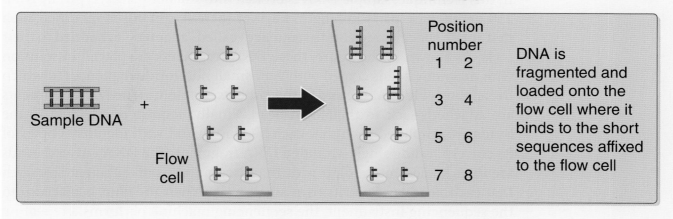

Position number
1 2
3 4
5 6
7 8

DNA is fragmented and loaded onto the flow cell where it binds to the short sequences affixed to the flow cell

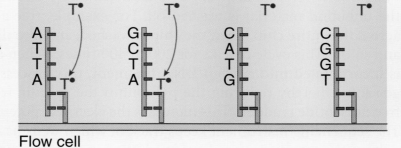

Sample DNA fragments

When T is flowed across the flow cell, it binds where A is in the first open template position

Cycle repeats flowing A, T, C, then G until all fragments have had complements built

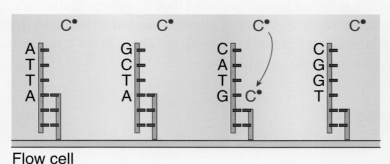

When C is flowed across the flow cell, it binds where G is in the first open template position

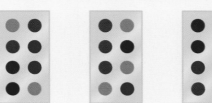

At each timepoint, colors and coordinates are used to reconstruct the order of incorporated bases for each fragment in parallel

Position number
1 2
3 4
5 6
7 8

Cycle 1   Cycle 2...   Cycle n

T: Red
C: Blue
A: Green
G: Orange

NEXT-GENERATION SEQUENCING SHORT READ: SEMICONDUCTOR SEQUENCING METHOD

In this technique, sample DNA is broken into smaller pieces, typically from 250 to 500 base pairs in length. Each of these fragments is modified such that small, specific nucleotide sequences called "adapters" are added to their ends. As shown in the figure, these DNA fragments are placed in solution with magnetic beads coated with very small nucleotide sequences to which the adapters bind. At the end of this process, single, unique DNA fragments are attached, each to their own bead. Finally, sequences attached to the beads are amplified such that each bead is coated with identical copies of its corresponding single-stranded DNA fragment. The DNA covered beads are then loaded into a chip with microscopic wells of sufficient size such that each bead lands in its own small well. When the chip is placed into the sequencing instrument, the sequencing machine performs a repeating cycle wherein free nucleotides are added to the chip one at a time, and then the unbound material is washed off. For example, free adenine is added across the entire chip. Then the chip is washed, and free thymine is added, and so on. This cycle repeats for 200 to 400 times. When a free nucleotide is incorporated into a given DNA fragment, this process releases hydrogen ions, thereby reducing the pH within the specific well in which the free nucleotide is added. This increases the electrical potential for that well. The sequencing instrument keeps track of which wells have had measured voltage changes during nucleotide addition, and converts that information into a series of bases for each DNA fragment added to the chip. This differs notably from sequencing by other manufacturers, in that nucleotide detection is electrical, and not optical. There is no camera required within the semiconductor instrument.

Next generation sequencing, short read: semiconductor sequencing method

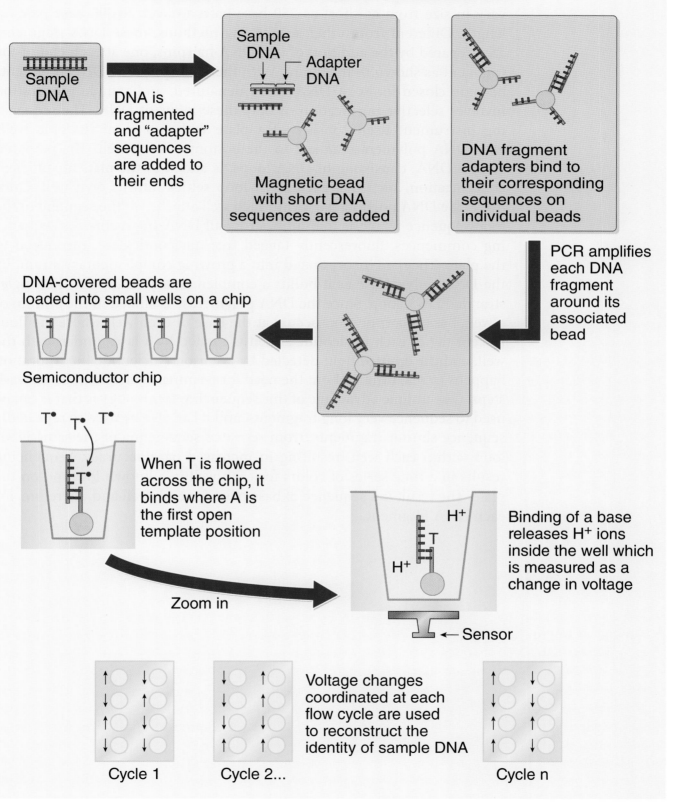

NEXT-GENERATION SEQUENCING LONG READ: SINGLE-MOLECULE REAL-TIME SEQUENCING METHOD

In this technique, sample DNA is broken into fragments which can vary in size from as short as 250 base pairs to over 20,000 base pairs in length. Different from other sequencing methods, these DNA fragments are prepared by the addition of two DNA hairpins, one at each end of the fragment as shown in the figure. With these hairpins, the DNA fragments become closed loops of DNA when denatured, and sample preparation involves selective purification of only these loops of DNA. The sequencing instrument itself consists of a plate with many microscopic wells with DNA polymerase affixed to the bottom of each well. The prepared sample DNA, consisting of DNA loops, is added to the plate at sufficient concentration, such that each DNA loop settles into its own well. Once there, the DNA polymerase within each well attaches to the segment of the loop sequence which is the same across all DNA fragments. As sequencing commences, fluorescently tagged free nucleotides are introduced to the plate. They are incorporated into a growing complementary strand by the DNA polymerase as it builds a complementary strand for the single-stranded DNA loop. Since the DNA polymerase is affixed to the bottom of a well, base incorporation occurs at the base of each well where the fluorescent tag of each nucleotide added is excited by a laser underneath the well, and the emitted light detected by a sensor. Nucleotide incorporation happens in real time without the need for terminating nucleotides or wash steps. One unique advantage of this sequencing technology is that it can be used to sequence very long fragments, and it can also be used to repeatedly sequence shorter fragments, from repeated sequencing of the same DNA loop within each well, resulting in increased base accuracy. Sequencing results in a time series of colors for each well in a known location on the plate. The result is a sequence of base pairs for each well and, therefore, for each DNA fragment.

Next generation sequencing, long read: single molecule real time sequencing

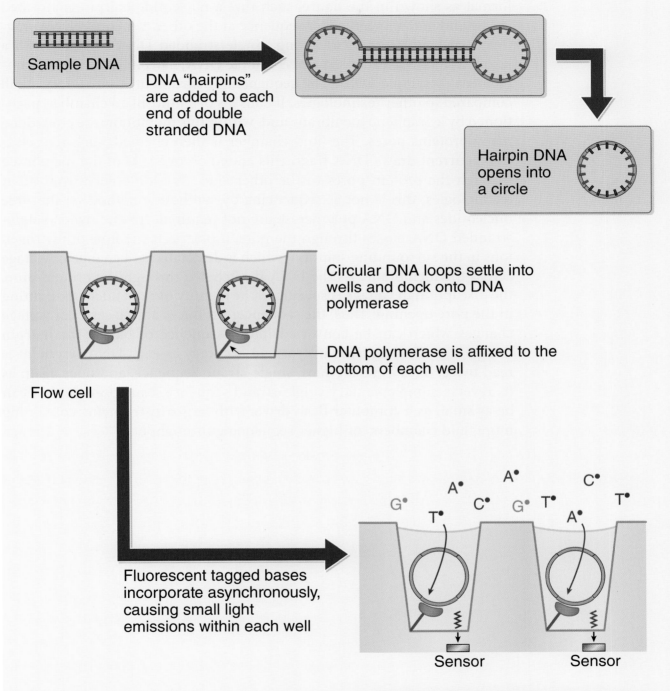

Sample DNA

DNA "hairpins" are added to each end of double stranded DNA

Hairpin DNA opens into a circle

Flow cell

Circular DNA loops settle into wells and dock onto DNA polymerase

DNA polymerase is affixed to the bottom of each well

Fluorescent tagged bases incorporate asynchronously, causing small light emissions within each well

Sensor   Sensor

Light emissions are recorded over time for each well and are used to reconstruct DNA sequences

NEXT-GENERATION SEQUENCING LONG READ: STRAND SEQUENCING PROTEIN NANOPORE METHOD

In this method, sample DNA is fragmented to produce long DNA pieces. These double-stranded fragments are then prepared in a "leader-hairpin" format as shown in the figure, such that a nucleotide hairpin is attached at one end and a linear leader sequence at the other. When the DNA fragments melt, this produces a long, single-stranded DNA segment with a layout as follows: leader sequence, sample DNA, hairpin, and reverse complement to sample DNA. The sequencing instrument itself is very small compared to other technologies. It consists of a fluid-filled chamber, partitioned by a graphene membrane and, within this membrane are embedded many proteins pores. The fluid chamber is then charged, such that electrical current draws DNA fragments added on one side of the membrane through the protein pores to the other side. As a difference from other technologies, this is not a "sequencing by synthesis" method, in that free nucleotides and DNA polymerase are not required. Instead, when single-stranded DNA passes through the pore, it obstructs the flow of hydrogen ions in the surrounding solution, which is detectable as a change in voltage across the membrane. As the DNA is ratcheted through the protein pore, the disruption in voltage is specific to the identity of each nucleotide sitting in the pore opening. Thus, the sequencer produces a time series of voltage changes which can be converted into a sequence of bases. The hairpin design is used to increase instrument accuracy as each DNA fragment is read twice, once as its forward, single-strand sequence, and once again as its reverse complementary single-strand sequence. Nanopore devices can be as small as a computer flash drive, with larger instruments containing more fluid chambers for higher sequencing throughput.

Next generation sequencing, long read: protein nanopore method

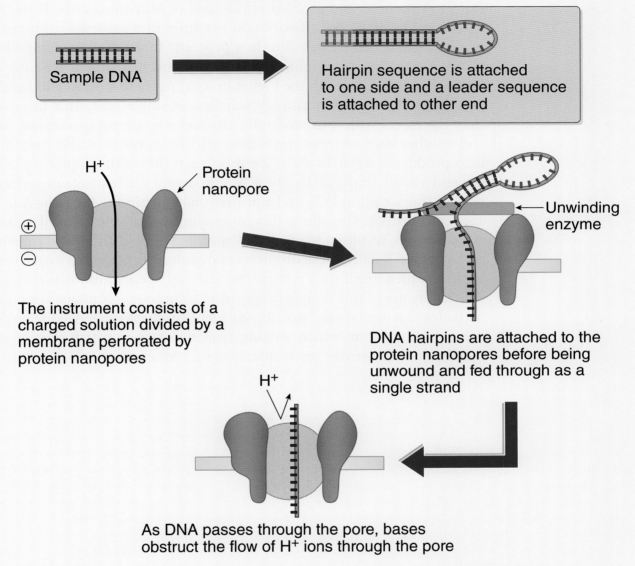

Sample DNA

Hairpin sequence is attached to one side and a leader sequence is attached to other end

H⁺

Protein nanopore

The instrument consists of a charged solution divided by a membrane perforated by protein nanopores

Unwinding enzyme

DNA hairpins are attached to the protein nanopores before being unwound and fed through as a single strand

H⁺

As DNA passes through the pore, bases obstruct the flow of H⁺ ions through the pore

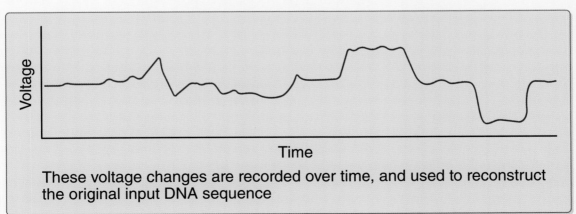

These voltage changes are recorded over time, and used to reconstruct the original input DNA sequence

NEXT-GENERATION SEQUENCING SINGLE-CELL TRANSCRIPTOMICS: "10× GENOMICS" METHOD

In this method, single cells are isolated such that their respective RNA can be sequenced and profiled at the level of individual cells. First tissue specimens undergo cell dissociation resulting in a suspension comprised of single cells. This suspension then proceeds through sequencing library preparation using a specialized instrument. This instrument is a microfluidic device (as pictured in the Figure on next page) that dilutes and isolates an input cell suspension into a linear flow of single cells. This linear flow then intersects with a microfluidic channel containing specialized beads and another such channel containing oil. The purpose of this instrument is to produce a water-in-oil suspension such that each droplet contains a cell and a bead. Importantly, these beads contain the requisite materials for reverse transcription PCR and a primer that will bind to the poly-A tail on each cell's mRNA. This allows this entire sample of droplets to undergo PCR amplification, resulting in small cell-specific RT-PCR amplification within each droplet. Finally, these droplets are dissolved and homogenized, resulting in a sequencing library compatible with next-generation sequencing but which—by use of this sample preparation technique—contains sequencing barcodes that can be used to uniquely identify which sequenced DNA fragments resulted from which starting droplet (i.e. from which starting cell), thereby enabling single-cell transcriptomic sequencing.

Next generation sequencing, synthetic long read: "10X genomics" method

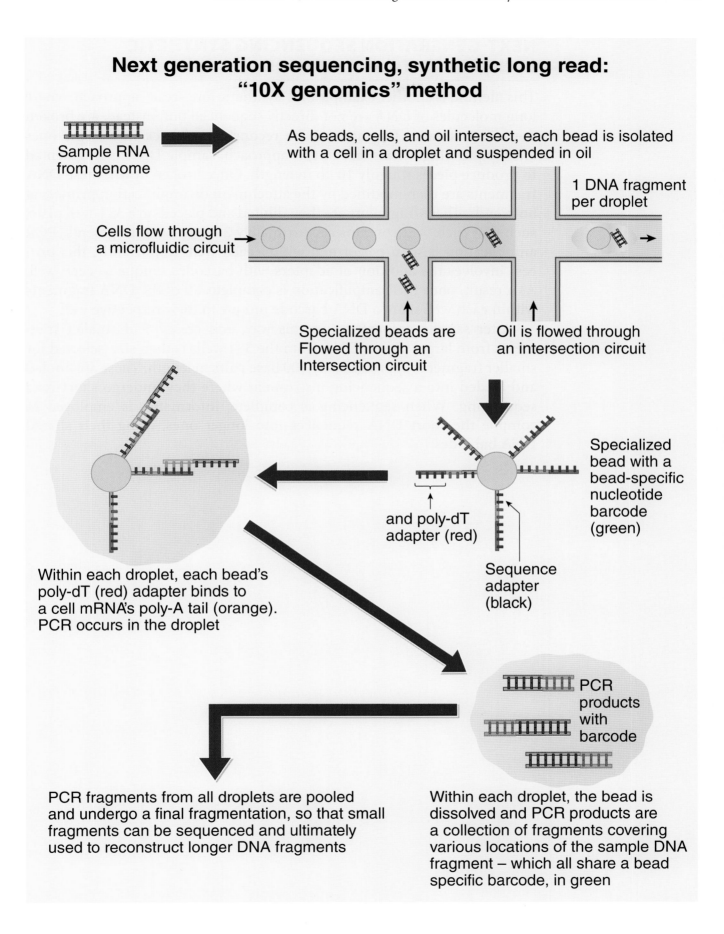

Sample RNA from genome

As beads, cells, and oil intersect, each bead is isolated with a cell in a droplet and suspended in oil

1 DNA fragment per droplet

Cells flow through a microfluidic circuit

Specialized beads are Flowed through an Intersection circuit

Oil is flowed through an intersection circuit

Specialized bead with a bead-specific nucleotide barcode (green)

and poly-dT adapter (red)

Sequence adapter (black)

Within each droplet, each bead's poly-dT (red) adapter binds to a cell mRNA's poly-A tail (orange). PCR occurs in the droplet

PCR products with barcode

PCR fragments from all droplets are pooled and undergo a final fragmentation, so that small fragments can be sequenced and ultimately used to reconstruct longer DNA fragments

Within each droplet, the bead is dissolved and PCR products are a collection of fragments covering various locations of the sample DNA fragment – which all share a bead specific barcode, in green

NEXT-GENERATION SEQUENCING SYNTHETIC LONG READ: "TRuSEQ" METHOD

This method is another example of a "synthetic long-read" approach, where long molecules of DNA are not directly sequenced but, instead, are broken down into smaller fragments to be reconstructed back into larger ones after sequencing is finished. In this approach, sample DNA is fragmented to produce pieces roughly 10 kb in length. Once broken down, these DNA fragments are then modified by the attachment of amplification primers at both ends. These fragments are then diluted and placed on a 384-well plate, such that each well contains approximately 3000 to 6000 fragments. PCR amplification is then performed within each well. Importantly, this process involves the addition of adapters with barcodes unique to each well. As a result, once PCR amplification is complete, all of the DNA fragments within each well share a DNA barcode unique to their respective well.

After sample preparation in this way, and creation of smaller fragments from larger pieces, DNA from the 384 wells is then size-selected for smaller fragments approximately 400 base pairs in length. These are pooled and loaded into a sequencing instrument where they undergo short-read sequencing. When sequencing is complete, informatics is employed to compile the short DNA sequences into longer ones, using their shared DNA barcodes.

Next generation sequencing, synthetic long read: TruSeq

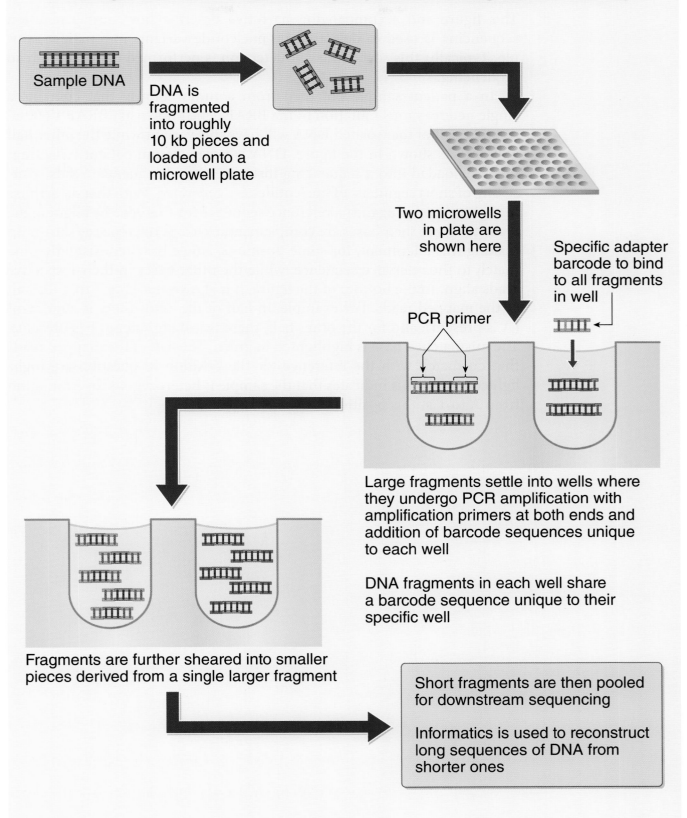

Sample DNA

DNA is fragmented into roughly 10 kb pieces and loaded onto a microwell plate

Two microwells in plate are shown here

Specific adapter barcode to bind to all fragments in well

PCR primer

Large fragments settle into wells where they undergo PCR amplification with amplification primers at both ends and addition of barcode sequences unique to each well

DNA fragments in each well share a barcode sequence unique to their specific well

Fragments are further sheared into smaller pieces derived from a single larger fragment

Short fragments are then pooled for downstream sequencing

Informatics is used to reconstruct long sequences of DNA from shorter ones

DETECTION OF A GENETIC ALTERATION USING NEXT-GENERATION SEQUENCING METHOD

This figure and accompanying narrative describe how next-generation sequencing is used to detect single-nucleotide variants in a patient sample. Typically, this sort of variant detection is performed using short-read sequencing.

In a patient sample obtained from a tumor biopsy that contains a single heterozygous mutation in the BRAF gene known as "BRAF V600E," roughly half of the isolated DNA will have this variant while the other half will not. As shown in the figure, DNA is isolated from patient cells, fragmented, loaded into a sequencing instrument, and sequence "reads" consisting of short segments of nucleotides are generated. With that data, those reads are mapped against a reference sequence for this gene by aligning the reads to where their bases are complementary to the reference as shown. In making this alignment, for some positions, single bases consistently mismatch to the reference sequence, while the other bases in their respective reads align. In the bottom of the figure, it is shown that this is true for half of the mapped reads. For example, in half of the reads there is alignment (A is present), and for the other half, there is misalignment (T is present). The mismatched base is highlighted in green. The half of the mapped reads that do match with the reference for the position in question are highlighted in red. This indicates that the sample is heterozygous for a mutation from A to T at this position in the BRAF gene.

Detection of a genomic alteration using next generation sequencing

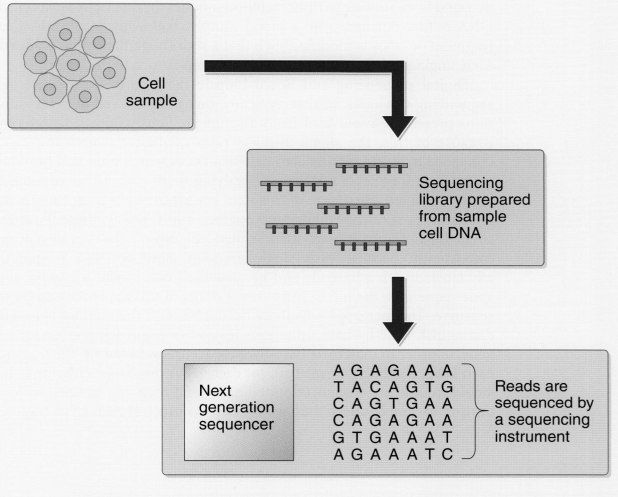

DIGITAL SEQUENCING

In a departure from other sequencing methods, digital sequencing is a technique aimed at maximizing sensitivity. It is essential to techniques such as a "liquid biopsy" where small amounts of circulating tumor DNA can be detected from routine peripheral blood samples. In this technique, cell-free DNA is first purified from a blood sample. Following purification, each fragment of DNA is modified such that a short oligonucleotide is added to each single-stranded half of each fragment as shown in the figure.

Digital sequencing and liquid biopsies also differ from some other sequencing use cases, in that, typically, this assay is used to detect mutations present at a low level from a set of previously known target genes. Because of this, the signal-to-noise ratio of digital sequencing can be enhanced by using biotinylated bait sequences which bind and pull down target gene fragments selectively, purifying them within the solution. For a more detailed discussion of this step, review the hybrid capture method described previously. Following preparation in this way, these libraries of small DNA fragments are then sequenced using a short-read platform. Importantly, because each single-stranded piece of DNA is individually labeled with a barcode and because the assay targets a specific set of gene sequences, the informatics components of this approach can be very sensitive. The increased sensitivity occurs because the method is tuned to distinguish base-by-base mutations instead of sequencing error for each gene, in order to maximize base-by-base accuracy. Secondly, the tagging of each DNA fragment means that, for each DNA piece in each sample, both single strands are sequenced individually and then can be used for comparison to double-check the base-by-base accuracy of each DNA fragment.

Digital sequencing

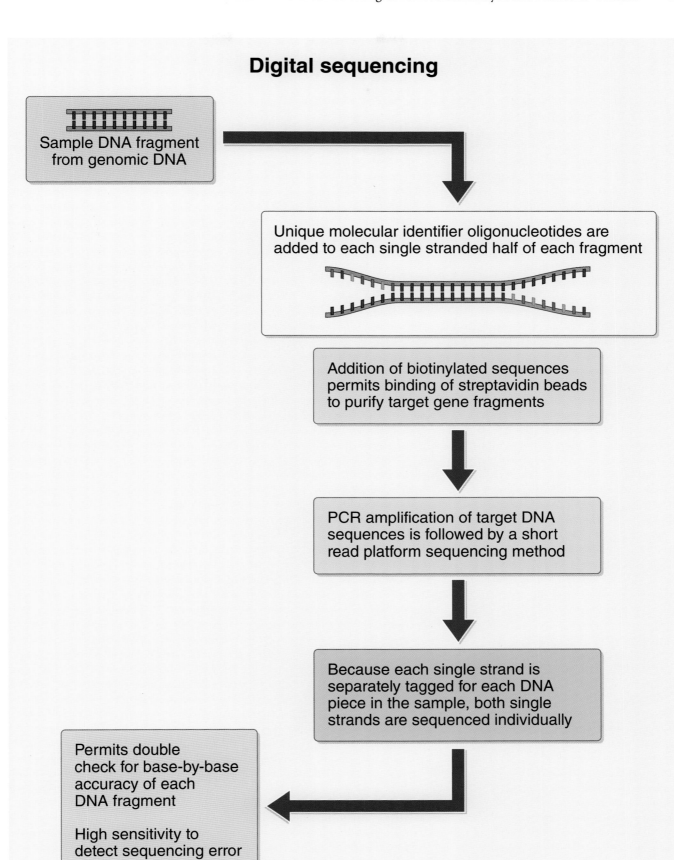

Sample DNA fragment from genomic DNA

Unique molecular identifier oligonucleotides are added to each single stranded half of each fragment

Addition of biotinylated sequences permits binding of streptavidin beads to purify target gene fragments

PCR amplification of target DNA sequences is followed by a short read platform sequencing method

Because each single strand is separately tagged for each DNA piece in the sample, both single strands are sequenced individually

Permits double check for base-by-base accuracy of each DNA fragment

High sensitivity to detect sequencing error

Self-Assessment Questions

1. What is the name of the test based on the following description of the methodology?
   Cells on glass slides are incubated with a patient's serum. Antibody is detected as present by adding fluorescent-labeled anti-IgG antibodies. Fluorescence staining of the nucleus of the cells on the glass slide can be homogeneous, rimmed, speckled, or nucleolar.
   - **A.** Serum protein electrophoresis
   - **B.** Antinuclear antibody (ANA) testing
   - **C.** Immunofixation electrophoresis
   - **D.** Flow cytometry

2. Which of the following parameters of a protein is least likely to affect its migration in protein electrophoresis?
   - **A.** Charge
   - **B.** Biological Function
   - **C.** Size
   - **D.** Shape

3. What is the name of the test based on the following description of the methodology? Patient serum or urine is added to lanes on an agarose gel, and the proteins are separated by electrophoresis. Antibodies are added on top of each individual lane with specificity for the immunoglobulin heavy chains, mu, gamma, and alpha, and the immunoglobulin light chains, kappa and lambda.
   - **A.** Serum protein electrophoresis
   - **B.** Antinuclear antibody (ANA) testing
   - **C.** Immunofixation electrophoresis
   - **D.** Flow cytometry

4. Which of the following methods is used to isolate a population of cells with a known cell surface antigen?
   - **A.** Flow cytometry
   - **B.** Electrophoresis
   - **C.** Nephelometry
   - **D.** Liquid chromatography

5. A 48-year-old woman with long-standing autoimmune disease has a blood sample collected into a heparin-containing vacuum tube. Shortly after the blood is collected into the tube, a precipitate forms that is noticeable upon observation with the naked eye. A second sample is collected. Which of the following forms of transportation of the sample to the clinical laboratory is least likely to prevent a precipitate from forming in the second tube?
   - **A.** Placement of the tube in warm sand at 37 °C with transportation to the laboratory
   - **B.** Transporting the sample along with STAT specimens at room temperature
   - **C.** Placement of the tube in water heated to 37 °C with transportation to the laboratory
   - **D.** Placement of the sample into a plastic bag carried to the laboratory under the arm of the transporter

6. A 65-year-old man with fever and dysuria provides a urine sample, and a Gram stain is performed. Rod-shaped bacteria are observed in high quantity. The Gram stain indicates the presence of which of the following pathogens?
   - **A.** Gram-positive streptococci
   - **B.** Gram-negative bacilli
   - **C.** Gram-negative diplococci
   - **D.** Gram-positive staphylococci

7. There are a variety of different agar plates used to promote the growth of bacteria. The need for different solid medium relates to which one of the following?
   A. There are different nutrients in the different agar plates to promote the selective growth of certain types of bacteria.
   B. Specific types of solid media are necessary to support the growth of viruses and parasites.
   C. The different colors of the solid media provide a background which makes small and clear colonies more visible.
   D. The use of certain types of solid media is intended to inhibit the growth of nonpathogenic bacteria.

8. Which of the following compounds is commonly used in the detection of a positive blood culture?
   A. Carbon dioxide
   B. Oxygen
   C. Nitrogen
   D. Hydrogen

9. In a test for antimicrobial sensitivity of a pathogenic organism on an agar plate using the disk diffusion method, the following diameters with no growth of microorganisms were obtained for the drugs noted. Which of the following drugs is most likely to be effective against the organism identified as pathogenic?
   A. Penicillin, 2 mm
   B. Clindamycin, 5 mm
   C. Vancomycin, 10 mm
   D. Clarithromycin, 25 mm

10. Which one of the following statements is true in the indirect immunofluorescence assay for antigen detection in a specimen applied onto a glass slide?
   A. A fluorescent-labeled antibody is used to bind to the antigen of interest on a glass slide.
   B. A second antibody directed at IgG and not conjugated to a fluorescent label is used as a reagent in the assay.
   C. A fluorescent antibody directed against unlabeled antibody binds to the antigen of interest on the glass slide to produce immunofluorescence.

D. Two fluorescent antibodies are required, producing red and green colors, with antigen detection.

11. In the automated blood cell counter, which of the following is a calculated value that is not measured directly by the instrument?
   A. Platelet count
   B. Hemoglobin
   C. White blood cell count
   D. Mean corpuscular hemoglobin concentration (MCHC)

12. Which of the following is not able to be determined in the review of a peripheral blood smear?
   A. Identification of separate B cell and T cell lymphocytes
   B. An approximation of the platelet count
   C. The size and shape of red blood cells
   D. Identification of immature white blood cells

13. Which of the following hemoglobin types will produce a negative screening test for sickle cell hemoglobin?
   A. Hemoglobin SC
   B. Hemoglobin SS
   C. Hemoglobin SA
   D. Hemoglobin CC

14. Which of the following hemoglobins is the least commonly identified hemoglobin by hemoglobin analysis in the US population?
   A. Hemoglobin S
   B. Hemoglobin C
   C. Hemoglobin A
   D. Hemoglobin G

15. The erythrocyte sedimentation rate has been a longstanding test to measure inflammation. Which of the following tests is also used as a marker of inflammation?
   A. Albumin
   B. Ceruloplasmin
   C. C-reactive protein (CRP)
   D. Immunoglobulin M

16. What is the unit of measurement for the PT and PTT assays?
   A. mg/dL
   B. Seconds
   C. Units/L
   D. nmol/L

17. Which set of test results is most consistent with the presence of a factor VIII inhibitor in a PTT mixing study at time points 0 hours (immediately), 30 minutes, and 1 hour after mixing?
    A. 60 seconds, 35 seconds, 58 seconds
    B. 60 seconds, 62 seconds, 58 seconds
    C. 60 seconds, 32 seconds, 30 seconds
    D. 60 seconds, 25 seconds, 28 seconds

18. Which of the following results are most likely to represent a coagulation factor VIII deficiency in a mixing study, in the absence of a coagulation factor VIII inhibitor?
    A. PTT prior to mixing with normal plasma is markedly prolonged 65 seconds; PTT after mixing for 30 minutes is normal at 28 seconds; PTT after 60 minutes remains normal at 30 seconds.
    B. PTT prior to mixing with normal plasma is markedly prolonged 65 seconds; PTT after mixing for 30 minutes is prolonged at 61 seconds; PTT after 60 minutes remains prolonged at 64 seconds.
    C. PTT prior to mixing with normal plasma is markedly prolonged 65 seconds; PTT after mixing for 30 minutes is slightly elevated at 38 seconds; PTT after 60 minutes is markedly prolonged at 72 seconds.
    D. PTT prior to mixing with normal plasma is normal at 30 seconds; PTT after mixing for 30 minutes is normal at 28 seconds; PTT after 60 minutes remains normal at 30 seconds.

19. Which of the following assays provides a quantitative measurement of von Willebrand activity?
    A. An immunoassay for von Willebrand factor protein
    B. An assay for coagulation factor VIII with clot detection
    C. A test that measures the ability of von Willebrand factor and ristocetin to promote platelet aggregation
    D. An antigenic assay for coagulation factor VIII

20. Which of the following is measured in a platelet aggregation assay?
    A. The ability of platelets to aggregate in response to platelet-activating agents
    B. The ability of platelets to bind to white blood cells in response to platelet-activating agents
    C. The ability of platelets to remain in suspension without aggregation in response to platelet-activating agents
    D. The ability of platelets to induce red cell clumping and hemolysis in response to platelet-activating agents

21. Which of the statements about blood typing is true?
    A. Forward typing detects antibodies in the serum that can bind to red blood cell antigens.
    B. Reverse typing detects antigens that bound to the red blood cell.
    C. In forward typing, antibodies to A, B, and Rh antigens are added to three separate tubes containing red blood cells.
    D. The failure of red blood cells to clump upon addition of antibodies to the A antigen indicates the presence of A antigen on red blood cells.

22. Which of the following statements about storage of blood components is correct?
    A. Packed red blood cells are stored at 20–24 °C.
    B. Platelet concentrates are stored at 1–6 °C.
    C. Plasma is stored at −18 °C (i.e., at least 18° below 0 °C).
    D. Whole blood is stored at below 18 °C.

23. Which one of the following is the correct combination in a blood cross match to determine the suitability of a donated red blood cell product for a potential recipient?
    A. Patient serum mixed with potential donor red blood cells
    B. Donor serum mixed with patient red blood cells
    C. Patient serum mixed with potential donor serum
    D. Patient red blood cells mixed with potential donor red blood cells

24. What is the name of the test that determines if immunoglobulin G (IgG) or complement component C3d is bound to a patient's red blood cells?
    A. The blood crossmatch
    B. The indirect antiglobulin test
    C. Red blood cell antigen detection test to identify antibodies to red blood cells
    D. The direct antiglobulin test

25. The goal of the indirect antiglobulin test is which of the following?

- **A.** Detect antibodies on the red blood cell surface.
- **B.** Detect antibodies in the plasma which can bind, but are not bound to red blood cells.
- **C.** Detect C3d in the plasma of the patient not bound to red blood cells.
- **D.** Detect C3d on the red blood cell surface.

26. Which one of the following compounds cannot be selectively removed by apheresis?

- **A.** Plasma
- **B.** Platelets
- **C.** Albumin
- **D.** White blood cells

27. Identification of antibodies to HIV antigens can be detected by which of the following assays?

- **A.** Western blot
- **B.** Indirect antiglobulin test
- **C.** Protein electrophoresis
- **D.** Indirect immunofluorescence

28. The measurement of the electrolytes in serum or plasma is most commonly performed using which of the following?

- **A.** Ion-selective electrode
- **B.** Spectrophotometer
- **C.** Mass spectrometer
- **D.** Gas chromatograph

29. Linked enzyme reactions to measure a compound or an enzyme activity in plasma, which generate a color change proportional to the concentration of the compound, are most commonly characterized by which one of the following?

- **A.** Highly automated and relatively inexpensive to perform
- **B.** Manual tests and relatively inexpensive to perform
- **C.** Highly automated and expensive to perform
- **D.** Manual tests and expensive to perform

30. The sample most commonly used for blood gas testing is which one of the following?

- **A.** Venous whole blood
- **B.** Serum
- **C.** Arterial whole blood
- **D.** Arterial plasma

31. Which of the following is detected by analysis of the sediment from a centrifuged urine specimen?

- **A.** Specific gravity
- **B.** Red blood cell casts
- **C.** Bilirubin
- **D.** Urobilinogen

32. What is the name of the test based on the following description of the methodology? A sample of acellular body fluid is incubated with an antibody to the compound being measured. When the compound is present, antigen–antibody complexes form, which scatter light from a beam of light shone through the sample. The amount of scattered light is proportional to the compound being measured.

- **A.** Flow cytometry for identification of cell type
- **B.** Cryoglobulin analysis
- **C.** Nephelometry for quantitation of proteins
- **D.** Immunofixation electrophoresis

33. D-dimers can be quantitated most precisely by which one of the following assays?

- **A.** Nephelometry
- **B.** Latex agglutination
- **C.** Western blot
- **D.** ELISA

34. Which of the following tests is a competitive binding assay?

- **A.** Latex agglutination
- **B.** Western blot
- **C.** ELISA without antigen or antibody fixed to a surface
- **D.** Platelet aggregation

35. A positive test in a latex agglutination assay is reported in what units?

- **A.** Nanograms per deciliter
- **B.** The highest dilution of the patient's specimen which produces agglutination
- **C.** Optical density
- **D.** The lowest dilution of the patient's specimen which produces agglutination

36. Which of the following statements is true regarding gas chromatography?

    A. Volatile compounds separated with gas as a mobile phase

    B. Volatile compounds separated with liquid as a mobile phase

    C. Nonvolatile compounds separated with gas as a mobile phase

    D. Nonvolatile compounds separated with liquid as a mobile phase

37. When molecular compounds are separated by liquid or gas chromatography and then the molecules are broken into different size fragments creating a "fingerprint" for each molecule, which of the following detectors is used?

    A. Spectrophotometer

    B. Ion-selective electrode

    C. Flame ionization detector

    D. Mass spectrometer

38. The sample used for a newborn screening test for inherited diseases is which of the following?

    A. Whole blood from a puncture of the skin

    B. Whole blood obtained from a vein

    C. Urine

    D. Sweat

39. Which of the following point-of-care tests is used more than the others?

    A. International normalized ratio (INR)

    B. Blood glucose

    C. Troponin

    D. Hemoglobin A1c

40. A pregnancy point-of-care test using urine as a test sample involves all but one of the following.

    A. Lateral flow of liquid to permit separation of compounds along a test strip

    B. Antibody capture of human chorionic gonadotropin (hCG)

    C. A control band on the strip to indicate a valid assay result

    D. Fluorescent detection of an antibody–hCG complex

41. Which of the following describes the evaluation of chromosomes by performance of a karyotype?

    A. Chromosomal analysis for structural abnormalities and abnormal number of chromosomes

    B. Total genome sequencing of an individual chromosome

    C. Identification of single-nucleotide variations

    D. Sequencing of an individual gene on a chromosome

42. Which of the following methods is commonly used to detect chromosomal rearrangements?

    A. Next-generation sequencing

    B. Serum protein electrophoresis

    C. Comparative genomic hybridization

    D. Fluorescence in situ hybridization

43. What is the primary function of polymerase chain reaction (PCR)?

    A. Detecting mutations in DNA

    B. Identifying chromosomal deletions

    C. Generating multiple copies of a given piece of DNA

    D. Producing antibodies

44. What best describes how PCR is used to detect genetic mutations?

    A. Mutated DNA is longer than nonmutated DNA and this is evident on a gel.

    B. Mutated DNA is always more negatively charged than normal DNA.

    C. Mutations occurring in places where normal primers bind will prevent or slow amplification.

    D. PCR is used to prepare DNA for flow cytometry.

45. Which of the following is true of RT-PCR?

    A. RT-PCR stands for RNA-Targeted PCR.

    B. RT-PCR turns RNA into complementary DNA before PCR amplification.

    C. RT-PCR uses PCR to detect antibody binding to sample DNA.

    D. RT-PCR turns DNA into complementary RNA before PCR amplification.

46. In what way is qPCR "Quantitative"?
    A. qPCR measures the abundance of a given sequence as the amount of fluorescence after repeated cycles of amplification.
    B. qPCR measures the mass spectra of sample DNA as a number.
    C. qPCR measures the quantity of hydrogen ions present in a blood sample.
    D. qPCR stands for "quick PCR" and so it reduces the quantity of time required for PCR.

47. Which of the following might be a good use case for DNA microarray?
    A. Detection of several mutations simultaneously in a given sample
    B. Detection of cancer-specific antibodies in a blood sample
    C. Sequencing of a novel genome that has never been sequenced before
    D. Determination of concentration of DNA in a library preparation for sequencing

48. Which of the following is NOT true about comparative genomic hybridization (CGH)?
    A. CGH only requires a sample DNA.
    B. CGH must have both sample DNA and a normal control DNA for comparison.
    C. CGH is generally used to detect chromosome rearrangements and not for single-point mutations.
    D. CGH can be performed using chromosomes or smaller target sequences arrayed on a chip.

49. Which of the following alterations is CGH generally best for detecting?
    A. Single-nucleotide variants
    B. Homopolymer runs
    C. Chromosomal rearrangements
    D. Deletion or duplication of chromosomal material

50. Hybrid capture is a technique best suited for which purpose?
    A. Amplifying a specific region of sample DNA
    B. Selecting a large subset of DNA from a sample such as an entire exome
    C. Selecting a small subset of DNA from a sample such as two key genes
    D. Attaching primers to DNA for sequencing

51. What best describes an amplicon?
    A. mRNA derived from a specific region of DNA
    B. A DNA or RNA segment that is the product of replication
    C. A DNA segment derived from RNA
    D. A DNA or RNA segment used to assess for the presence of insertions or deletions

52. Sanger sequencing uses what technique to determine the order of bases in a given sequence?
    A. Bases closer to the front of a target sequence are brighter and can be detected using a fluorescence detector.
    B. For a given target sequence, all sequences are ordered by size which is equivalent to ordering by length.
    C. Bases are color-coded according to their position in the original sequence with red bases always being in front.
    D. Sanger sequencing uses a semiconductor to detect bases.

53. What is the general tradeoff between short-read and long-read sequencing?
    A. Typically, shorter reads are more accurate at each base but harder to reconstruct into their original DNA sequence, while long reads are easier to reconstruct but less accurate at each base.
    B. Short reads take far less time to produce than long reads and are performed at increased cost.
    C. Short reads take far more time to produce than long reads and are performed at reduced cost.
    D. Short reads and long reads are terms used by different manufacturers for sequencing methods.

54. How does the semiconductor sequencing device detect the incorporation of a given base into a DNA fragment?
    A. It uses a mass detection device to measure the increase in mass in a DNA fragment following base incorporation.
    B. It uses a fluorescence detector to detect the release of base-specific fluorescent probes.
    C. It detects the change in voltage resulting from a base incorporation within a small well.
    D. It uses gel electrophoresis to sort DNA fragments in order of incorporated bases.

55. How is DNA packaged when it is being sequenced using the single molecule real time sequencing (SMRT) method?

   A. DNA is formed into a hairpin, allowing both forward and reverse complement strands to pass through a detector.

   B. DNA is circularized and each DNA loop is sequenced in a separate small well.

   C. DNA is fragmented into independent, single-stranded pieces and laid out across a glass slide.

   D. DNA is supercoiled to maximize density.

56. How are nucleotides identified using a nanopore instrument?

   A. Each base has a color-coded fluorescent tag, and when these are added as complementary to sample DNA, a fluorescence detector reads this color information.

   B. Each segment of sample DNA is directly measured as it passes through a protein channel.

   C. Each segment of sample DNA is run on an electrophoresis gel with size representing base identity.

   D. Each base has an antibody tag and, when these are added as complementary to sample DNA, an immunoassay is used to identify each base.

57. Which of the following best described how a 10× Genomics instrument performs single-cell sequencing?

   A. Each long DNA strand is directly sequenced on an instrument with a nanopore.

   B. Each cell is directly affixed to a microwell directly on an Illumina sequencing chip.

   C. Each cell is isolated into its own bubble where is undergoes amplification and incorporation of a unique, bubble-specific sequence before downstream sequencing.

   D. Each cell's nucleus is aggregated to undergo Sanger sequencing.

58. How does True Seq synthetic long-read technology differ from 10× genomics?

   A. TruSeq does not fragment long DNA strands.

   B. TruSeq does not use oil bubbles to isolate longer DNA fragments.

   C. TruSeq does not use PCR.

   D. TruSeq is not compatible with short-read sequencing.

59. Which of the following is necessary to using next-generation sequencing to detect single-nucleotide variants?

   A. Each variant corresponds to a separate location on an electrophoresis gel.

   B. Each variant is detected by microarray probes with different colors.

   C. Each variant is part of a read which is aligned to a reference gene sequence revealing mutations as mismatches to the reference.

   D. Each variant has a unique mass-to-charge ratio detectable on sequencing.

60. Which of the following is the best use case for consideration of digital sequencing?

   A. Detection of large structural rearrangements in tumor DNA

   B. Detection of long repeat sequences in microbial DNA

   C. Detection of copy number variation in tumor DNA

   D. Detection of low-abundance cell-free DNA in peripheral blood

Self-Assessment Answers

1. **The correct answer is B.** The test involving fixed cells on glass slides is the antinuclear antibody test.
2. **The correct answer is B.** Charge, size, and shape are physical characteristics of the protein which impact its migration in protein electrophoresis. The function of the protein, which could be an enzyme or a transport protein, for example, will not affect migration in an electrophoretic system.
3. **The correct answer is C.** The test involving an agarose gel and antibodies is immunofixation electrophoresis.
4. **The correct answer is A.** Flow cytometry is a test involving intact cells. The other methods involve molecules of different types.
5. **The correct answer is B.** This patient has a cryoglobulin which precipitates out of solution below 37 °C. The ineffective method is the one involving transport of the sample at room temperature which is well below 37 °C.
6. **The correct answer is B.** Bacilli are rod-shaped organisms, and red-colored bacteria in a Gram stain are gram negative.
7. **The correct answer is A.** Certain types of bacteria form colonies more effectively when specific nutrients are added into the semisolid agar. The presence or absence of certain compounds in the agar influences the color of the agar in the plate.
8. **The correct answer is A.** Carbon dioxide is generated by the growth of microorganisms in the blood culture bottles.
9. **The correct answer is D.** The larger the diameter that is organism free around an antibiotic disk, the more likely it is to be an effective drug to treat the infection. Organisms are reported as sensitive or resistant to an antibiotic based upon the diameter with no growth.
10. **The correct answer is C.** In the indirect immunofluorescence assay, it is only the second antibody which is bound to a fluorescent tag.
11. **The correct answer is D.** All other values are directly determined by the instrument.
12. **The correct answer is A.** Although lymphocytes can be identified in a peripheral blood smear, typing of lymphocytes as B cells or T cells is not possible when the blood smear is stained with Wright stain.
13. **The correct answer is D.** Screening tests for sickle cell hemoglobin require that at least one of the globin chains is altered from normal to produce sickle hemoglobin. Hemoglobin CC, therefore, while representing a hemoglobinopathy, would have a negative screening test for sickle hemoglobin.
14. **The correct answer is D.** The others are much more commonly encountered in the United States.
15. **The correct answer is C.** The others are not used as biomarkers of inflammation, even if their blood concentrations change in the presence of inflammation.
16. **The correct answer is B.** They are tests that measure the time until a clot forms in the sample after adding reagents to initiate clot formation.
17. **The correct answer is A.** It shows an immediate correction that prolongs at later time points. Choice B is most suggestive of a lupus anticoagulant. Choices C and D are most consistent with a PTT-related factor deficiency.
18. **The correct answer is D.** A coagulation factor deficiency is identified in this case as a PTT

mixing study with normal plasma that corrects into the reference range immediately upon mixing and stays in the reference range for an hour after mixing.

19. **The correct answer is C.** Choice A is an antigenic, not an activity, measurement of von Willebrand activity. Choice B refers to a measurement of Factor VIII activity, which is not von Willebrand factor. Choice D is an antigenic measurement of Factor VIII.

20. **The correct choice is A.** Platelet aggregation in platelet-rich plasma to a standard battery of agonists is the gold standard test for platelet function.

21. **The correct answer is C.** Forward typing detects antigens on red blood cells. Reverse typing detects antibodies that can bind to red blood cell antigens. Failure of red blood cells to clump in response to antibody indicates the absence of the corresponding antigen on the red blood cell.

22. **The correct answer is C.** Freshly collected plasma is stored frozen. Packed red blood cells are stored at 1–6 °C. Platelets are stored at 20–24 °C. Whole blood is stored at 1–6 °C.

23. **The correct choice is A.** The goal of the assay is to determine if a patient who requires a red blood cell transfusion has serum antibodies that can bind to donor red blood cells.

24. **The correct answer is D.** If IgG or C3d is present on the red blood cells, antibody to those proteins binds to the red blood cells, resulting in red blood cell agglutination and/or hemolysis.

25. **The correct choice is B.** The test to detect antibodies or C3d bound to red blood cells is the direct antiglobulin test. There is no clinical laboratory test directed at detection of C3d in the serum of a patient.

26. **The correct choice is C.** Apheresis can be used to remove plasma, but an individual protein in plasma, such as albumin, is not removable in a standard apheresis procedure.

27. **The correct choice is A.** Choice B relates to antibodies on red blood cells. Fluorescence is not involved in the detection of antibodies to HIV. Protein electrophoresis does not involve the use of antibodies.

28. **The correct answer is A.** The other devices are not used for electrolyte measurement.

29. **The correct answer is A.** These are the assays that are best suited to be performed on large automated analyzers and are relatively inexpensive.

30. **The correct answer is C.** An arterial whole blood sample is most commonly used for blood gas testing.

31. **The correct answer is B.** All the other measurements are performed on the liquid urine rather than the urine sediment, and the values are usually indicated by color changes on pads mounted on a urine dipstick.

32. **The correct answer is C.** The reason that it is not flow cytometry, used for identification of cell type, is that the sample being tested is acellular.

33. **The correct answer is D.** There is a test for D-dimers by latex agglutination but it is semi-quantitative. Nephelometry is not used to quantitate D-dimers. The data from a Western blot assay is qualitative (yes/no).

34. **The correct choice is C.** The initially developed ELISA tests involved capture antigen or capture antibody bound to the surface of a well. To allow for a simpler homogenous assay in which all reagents are in solution, an ELISA involving competitive binding was created.

35. **The correct answer is B.** There is a test for D-dimers by latex agglutination, but it is semi-quantitative with the result representing the highest dilution of the patient specimen that produces visible agglutination of the latex particles.

36. **The correct answer is A.** In a gas chromatograph, the temperature inside the instrument is very high, volatilizing the compounds which are being separated. The compounds are moved through the column toward the detector with a gaseous mobile phase, which is often helium.

37. **The correct answer is D.** The fragments of different masses create the molecular "fingerprint."

38. **The correct answer is A.** Typically a whole blood sample is obtained by puncturing the skin at the heel of a newborn. Blood from the puncture site is dripped onto a card, and tests are performed from blood eluted from the individual spots.

39. **The correct answer is B.** Among the four choices in this list, blood glucose is by far used

the most. Urine pregnancy point-of-care testing, which is not on this list, is also a commonly used assay, but not nearly as much as blood glucose.

40. **The correct answer is D.** Lateral flow of liquid along the test strip brings the hCG in the sample to the position where a line of antibodies that capture hCG are located on the strip, producing a visible band. There is a band on the strip which always appears in an assay which has valid result, whether the hCG band is present or not. The bands can be seen with the naked eye, and no fluorescence is required for detection.

41. **The correct answer is A.** The karyotype is a picture of full-length chromosomes captured in metaphase, to search for structural abnormalities or an abnormal number of chromosomes.

42. **The correct answer is D.** FISH is most commonly used to detect chromosomal rearrangements, and the location and proximity of fluorescent probes will indicate whether chromosomal locations have been altered. CGH is not used to detect chromosomal rearrangements. Next-generation sequencing is generally used to detect single-nucleotide variants, and serum protein electrophoresis is often used to detect the presence of monoclonal antibodies in serum.

43. **The correct answer is C.** The PCR is a very popular technique for amplifying DNA and uses the enzymatic action of DNA polymerase to synthesize DNA and make many copies of an initial DNA sample. This is a typical "upstream" technique for many testing assays as they require amplification of input DNA prior to testing.

44. **The correct answer is C.** PCR can be used in a variety of ways to help in the detection of mutations. However, from among the list of options, the only one that applied to PCR is C. The principle of the test is that primer sequences will bind to a DNA strand leading to the amplification of DNA in between primer sites. If there is a mutation in one of those sites and primer binding is inhibited, amplification will also be reduced or absent, and this is detectable in the assay.

45. **The correct answer is B.** RT-PCR stands for reverse transcription PCR and uses reverse transcriptase enzymes to convert RNA into cDNA before doing PCR amplification.

46. **The correct answer is A.** qPCR measures the abundance of fluorescence signal over several successive cycles of PCR amplification, and uses this to measure the abundance of starting material, "target DNA or RNA," in a given sample.

47. **The correct answer is A.** DNA microarrays can simultaneously detect multiple mutations occurring at different locations throughout a sample genome by creating a "lawn" of smaller DNA sequences known as "probes," representing several areas of interest within the genome and laying them out on a chip. Binding of sample DNA fragments to various probe sequences is measured as the presence and relative abundance of a given target sequence or mutation.

48. **The correct answer is A.** As the name suggests, CGH is a comparative technique and so it measures the relative abundance of chromosomal material between a given sample and a normal reference. This comparison is how it can detect the relative gain, loss, or equivalence of a given chromosomal area when compared to normal genomic material.

49. **The correct answer is D.** CGH lacks the resolution to detect single-nucleotide or multinucleotide features and is instead generally used to compare the abundance of chromosomal material in a given sample. Thus, this is best for detection deletions or duplications, known as "copy number variation."

50. **The correct answer is B.** Hybrid capture is an efficient technique for selecting many sequences from a sample. As such, it is typically used to filter for a large subset of an input sample, such as a whole exome. There are far too many sequences in all the exons to amplify them by PCR.

51. **The correct answer is B.** Amplicon sequencing is an efficient technique to selectively amplify a small subset of input DNA, such as a group of genes for downstream sequencing.

52. **The correct answer is B.** Sanger sequencing takes an input segment of DNA and builds many complementary strands each of which terminates at a different location in the target sequence. By ordering these strands by size,

which is equivalent to ordering them by length, the order of bases can be reconstructed and the identity of bases in that order can be determined by color-coded fluorescent tags.

53. **The correct answer is A.** Short-read sequencing is more accurate than long-read sequencing but can be very challenging when it comes to reconstructing original input DNA sequences, especially if those original sequences contain repeat regions. Long reads are easier to reconstruct, but they have limited accuracy, making such platforms not suitable for clinical testing for changes such as single-nucleotide variations.

54. **The correct answer is C.** The semiconductor sequencing device does not require a camera or fluorescence detector. Instead, it uses a semiconductor chip to which fragments of sample DNA are attached. When a given base is incorporated into a fragment of sample DNA, this releases hydrogen ions, resulting in a change in voltage detectable within the immediate vicinity of that DNA fragment. The voltage changes over time, and their coordinates on the semiconductor chip are used to reconstruct the DNA sequence of each fragment arrayed on the chip.

55. **The correct answer is B.** "Single Molecule Real-Time Sequencing" (SMRT) requires the creation of circular loops of DNA, after which each loop is sequenced within a specific small well by docking onto an immobilized DNA polymerase.

56. **The correct answer is B.** The nanopore instrument is not a sequence-by-synthesis device. Instead, it reads strands of sample DNA directly as they pass through a protein pore inserted into a membrane. Each specific nucleotide results in a specific voltage change at the pore, and these are converted back into a sequence of bases identified by the instrument's software.

57. **The correct answer is C.** Each cell is isolated into its own bubble wherein reverse transcription and PCR amplification occur. Since these processes are segregated into separate cell-specific bubbles, each gel bead containing PCR reagents also includes a unique nucleotide sequence (barcode) that gets incorporated upon PCR. Thus, when all bubbles are consolidated and sequenced, it is still possible to partition sequencing data according to each cell-specific barcode.

58. **The correct answer is B.** "TruSeq" Synthetic Long Read technology is similar in many ways to 10× Genomics linked-read sequencing, in that long DNA fragments are physically isolated into smaller pools where they undergo barcoding and amplification. Unlike 10× genomics, TruSeq does not isolate individual long DNA molecules into their own oil bubbles.

59. **The correct answer is C.** Detection of single-nucleotide variants using next-generation sequencing relies upon the creation of sequencing reads, some portion of which contain the variant of interest. As these are aligned to a reference sequence, for a known gene, these mutations appear as mismatched when compared to the reference. This is commonly known as read mapping, and can be useful in determining both the identity as well as the relative fraction of mutations among sample DNA.

60. **The correct answer is D.** Digital sequencing is a technique showing much promise in enabling the use of the "liquid biopsy," whereby cancerous mutations can be detected from peripheral blood. As such, this technique focuses on the recovery and detection of mutations present in trace amounts of circulating, cell-free DNA.

Further Reading

Bumgarner R. Overview of DNA microarrays: Types, applications, and their future. *Curr Protocols Mol Biol*. 2013;6137(suppl 101): 1-17. https://doi.org/10.1002/0471142727.mb2201s101

Carroll KC, Pfaller MA, Landry ML, et al., eds. *Manual of Clinical Microbiology*. 12th ed., Washington, DC: ASM Press; 2019.

Cui C, Shu W, Li P. Fluorescence in situ hybridization: Cell-based genetic diagnostic and research applications. *Front Cell Dev Biol*. 2016;4(Sep): 1-11. https://doi.org/10.3389/fcell.2016.00089

Deepak SA, Kottapalli KR, Rakwal R, et al. Real-time PCR: Revolutionizing detection and expression analysis of genes. *Curr Genom*. 2007;8(4):234-251. https://doi.org/10.2174/138920207781386960

Fung MK, Eder AE, Spitalnik SL, Westhoff CM, eds. *Technical Manual*. 19th ed. Bethesda, MD: AABB; 2017.

Garibyan L, Avashia N. Research techniques made simple: Polymerase chain reaction (PCR). *J Invest Dermatol*. 2013;133(3):1-4. https://doi.org/10.2807/ese.18.04.20382-en

Gaudin M, Desnues C. Hybrid capture-based next generation sequencing and its application to human infectious diseases. *Front Microbiol*. 2018;29(Nov):1-9. https://doi.org/10.3389/fmicb.2018.02924

Goodwin S, McPherson JD, McCombie WR. Coming of age: Ten years of next-generation sequencing technologies. *Nature Rev Gen*. 2016;17(6):333-351. Nature Publishing Group. https://doi.org/10.1038/nrg.2016.49

Head SR, Kiyomi Komori H, LaMere SA, et al. Library construction for next-generation sequencing: Overviews and challenges. *BioTechniques*. 2014;56(2):61-77. https://doi.org/10.2144/000114133

Heather JM, Chain B. The sequence of sequencers: The history of sequencing DNA. *Genomics*. 2016;107(1):1-8. Academic Press Inc. https://doi.org/10.1016/j.ygeno.2015.11.003

Kallioniem A, Kallioniemi O, Sudar D, et al. Comparative genomic hybridization for molecular cytogenetic analysis of solid tumors. *Science*. 1992;258:818-821.

Kaushansky K, Lichtman MA, Beutler E, Kipps TJ, Seligson U, Prchal JT, eds. *Williams Hematology*. 8th ed. New York: McGraw-Hill; 2010.

Kuleshov V, Xie D, Chen R, et al. Whole-genome haplotyping using long reads and statistical methods. *Nat Biotechnol*. 2014;32(3):261-266. https://doi.org/10.1038/nbt.2833

Lanman RB, Mortimer SA, Zil OA, et al. Analytical and clinical validation of a digital sequencing panel for quantitative, highly accurate evaluation of cell-free circulating tumor DNA. *PLoS ONE*. 2015;10(10):1-27. https://doi.org/10.1371/journal.pone.0140712

Laposata M, Connor AM, Hicks DG, Phillips DK. *The Clinical Hemostasis Handbook*. Chicago, IL: Year Book Medical Publishers Inc.; 1989.

McPherson RA, Pincus MR, eds. *Henry's Clinical Diagnosis and Management by Laboratory Methods*. 22nd ed. Philadelphia, PA: WB Saunders; 2017.

Ohan NW, Heikkila JJ. Reverse transcriptase—polymerase chain reaction: An overview of the technique and its applications. *Biotechnol Adv*. 1993;11(43):13-29.

Powers LW. Diagnostic Hematology: Clinical and Technical Principles. St. Louis, MO: The CV Mosby Company; 1989.

Rifai N, Horvath AR, Wittwer CT, eds. *Tietz Textbook of Clinical Chemistry and Molecular Diagnostics.* 6th ed. St. Louis, MO: Elsevier; 2018.

Simon TL, McCullough J, Snyder EL, Solheim BG, Strauss RG, eds. *Rossi's Principles of Transfusion Medicine.* 5th ed. West Sussex, UK: J Wiley & Sons; 2016.

Stites DP, Terr AI, Parslow TG, eds. *Basic and Clinical Immunology.* 8th ed. Norwalk, CT: Appleton & Lange; 1994.

Tille PM. *Bailey and Scott's Diagnostic Microbiology.* 13th ed. St. Louis, MO: Elsevier (Moseby); 2014.

Clinical Laboratory Reference Values

The conventional units in this table are the ones most commonly used in the United States. Outside the United States, SI units are the predominant nomenclature for laboratory test results. The base units in the SI system related to laboratory testing that are found in this table include the mole (amount of substance), meter (length), kilogram (mass), second (time), and Celsius (temperature).

Reference ranges vary depending on the instrument and the reagents used to perform the test. Therefore, the reference ranges shown in this table are only close approximations to the adult reference ranges found in an individual clinical laboratory. For example, coagulation tests measured in seconds until a clot forms in the tube, such as the PT and the PTT, have reference ranges that are affected by both the instrument and the reagents used to perform the test. There are more than 100 possible combinations of coagulation instruments and reagents, and, therefore, there are at least 100 different reference ranges, which are mostly similar but not identical. The cutoff value for troponin for acute myocardial infarction is at the 99th percentile of a reference range which is also instrument and reagent dependent. In addition, it is important to understand that reference ranges can be significantly affected by age and sex.

The table contains information about selected drugs for which there is no reference range because they are not present in the circulation of those not taking the drug. However, drugs which are monitored have therapeutic levels, and some of these are included in the list of reference ranges. The therapeutic range for a drug is most often established by the concentration of the drug just prior to administration of the next dose. This is called the trough level. For other drugs, the therapeutic range refers to its range at peak concentration. This varies from drug to drug and is dependent upon many factors, such as absorption, distribution within the body, and metabolism of the drug. The table does not indicate whether the therapeutic level is a peak or a trough level.

Also listed in the table are selected compounds which are neither drugs nor laboratory tests, but are compounds which can be measured in the blood and, at some concentration, become toxic. For these listings, the compound is named and the word (toxic) is listed on the same line.

Conversion factors are provided in the table to allow the reader to convert conventional units to SI units and vice versa. The conversion of the conventional unit to SI unit requires a multiplication with the conversion factor, and conversion of the SI unit to the conventional unit requires division by the conversion factor.

The sample fluid is sometimes highly restrictive. For example, coagulation tests must be performed using plasma samples. Serum samples are unacceptable. For other compounds, both plasma samples and serum samples may be acceptable. However, there may be differences, often minor, in the results obtained using plasma versus serum. Potassium is one such compound in which reference ranges may be different for plasma and serum. There is a significant movement away from the use of serum in favor of plasma. The principal reason for this is that extra time is required for samples to clot so that serum may be generated. A sample collected into a tube with an anticoagulant results in the generation of plasma rather than serum after the tube is centrifuged. The clotting step is omitted when plasma samples are prepared, and, therefore, the turnaround time for the performance of the test is shortened. In some circumstances, whole blood is used for analysis, but the number of tests performed using whole blood is very limited. Urine and other body fluids, such as pleural fluid and cerebrospinal fluid, are also used for testing. Some of the entries in the table are associated with a fluid other than plasma, serum, or whole blood.

	Specimen	Traditional Reference Interval	Traditional Units	Conversion Factor, Multiply →, ← Divide	SI Reference Interval	SI Units
Acetaminophen (therapeutic)	Serum, plasma	10–30	µg/mL	6.62	70–200	µmol/L
Acetoacetic acid	Serum, plasma	<1	mg/dL	0.098	<0.1	mmol/L
Acetone	Serum, plasma	<2.0	mg/dL	0.172	<0.34	mmol/L
Acetylcholinesterase	Red blood cells	5–10	U/mL	1	5–10	U/L
Activated partial thromboplastin time (APTT)	Whole blood	25–40	seconds	1	25–40	seconds
Adenosine deaminase[a]	Serum	11.5–25.0	U/L	0.017	0.20–0.43	µKat/L
Adrenocorticotropic hormone (ACTH) (see corticotropin)						
Alanine[b] (adult)	Plasma	1.87–5.88	mg/dL	112.2	210–661	µmol/day
Alanine aminotransferase (ALT, SGPT)[b]	Serum	10–40	U/L	1	10–40	U/L
Albumin[b]	Serum	3.5–5.0	g/dL	10	35–50	g/L
Alcohol (see ethanol, isopropanol, methanol)						
Alcohol dehydrogenase[a]	Serum	<2.8	U/L	0.017	<0.05	µKat/L
Aldolase[a,b]	Serum	1.0–7.5	U/L	0.017	0.02–0.13	µKat/L
Aldosterone[b] (upright)	Plasma	7–30	ng/dL	0.0277	0.19–0.83	nmol/L
Aldosterone	Urine, 24 h	3–20	µg/24 h	2.77	8–55	nmol/day
Alkaline phosphatase[b]	Serum	50–120	U/L	1	50–120	U/L
α_1-Acid glycoprotein	Serum	50–120	mg/dL	0.01	0.5–1.2	g/L
α_2-Macroglobulin	Serum	130–300	mg/dL	0.01	1.3–3.0	g/L
Alprazolam (therapeutic)	Serum, plasma	10–50	ng/mL	3.24	32–162	nmol/L
Aluminum	Serum, plasma	<6	ng/mL	37.06	0.0–222.4	nmol/L
Amikacin (therapeutic)	Serum, plasma	20–30	µg/mL	1.71	34–52	µmol/L
Amino acid fractionation:						
Alanine[b]	Plasma	1.87–5.89	mg/dL	112.2	210–661	µmol/L
α-Aminobutyric acid[b]	Plasma	0.08–0.36	mg/dL	97	8–35	µmol/L
Arginine[b]	Plasma	0.37–2.40	mg/dL	57.4	21–138	µmol/L
Asparagine[b]	Plasma	0.40–0.91	mg/dL	75.7	30–69	µmol/L
Aspartic acid[b]	Plasma	<0.3	mg/dL	75.1	<25	µmol/L
Citrulline[b]	Plasma	0.2–1.0	mg/dL	57.1	12–55	µmol/L
Cystine[b]	Plasma	0.40–1.40	mg/dL	83.3	33–117	µmol/L
Glutamic acid[b]	Plasma	0.2–2.8	mg/dL	67.97	15–190	µmol/L
Glutamine[b]	Plasma	6.1–10.2	mg/dL	68.42	420–700	µmol/L
Glycine[b]	Plasma	0.9–4.2	mg/dL	133.3	120–560	µmol/L
Histidine[b]	Plasma	0.5–1.7	mg/dL	64.5	32–110	µmol/L
Hydroxyproline[b]	Plasma	<0.55	mg/dL	76.3	<42	µmol/L
Isoleucine[b]	Plasma	0.5–1.3	mg/dL	76.24	40–100	µmol/L
Leucine[b]	Plasma	1.0–2.3	mg/dL	76.3	75–175	µmol/L
Lysine[b]	Plasma	1.2–3.5	mg/dL	68.5	80–240	µmol/L
Methionine[b]	Plasma	0.1–0.6	mg/dL	67.1	6–40	µmol/L

	Specimen	Traditional Reference Interval	Traditional Units	Conversion Factor, Multiply →, ← Divide	SI Reference Interval	SI Units
Ornithine[b]	Plasma	0.4–1.4	mg/dL	75.8	30–106	µmol/L
Phenylalanine[b]	Plasma	0.6–1.5	mg/dL	60.5	35–90	µmol/L
Proline[b]	Plasma	1.2–3.9	mg/dL	86.9	104–340	µmol/L
Serine[b]	Plasma	0.7–2.0	mg/dL	95.2	65–193	µmol/L
Taurine[b]	Plasma	0.3–2.1	mg/dL	80	24–168	µmol/L
Threonine[b]	Plasma	0.9–2.5	mg/dL	84	75–210	µmol/L
Tryptophan[b]	Plasma	0.5–1.5	mg/dL	48.97	25–73	µmol/L
Tyrosine[b]	Plasma	0.4–1.6	mg/dL	55.19	20–90	µmol/L
Valine[b]	Plasma	1.7–3.7	mg/dL	85.5	145–315	µmol/L
α-Aminobutyric acid[b]	Plasma	0.08–0.36	mg/dL	97	8–35	µmol/L
Amiodarone (therapeutic)	Serum, plasma	0.5–2.5	µg/mL	1.55	0.8–3.9	µmol/L
δ-Aminolevulinic acid	Urine	1.0–7.0	mg/24 h	7.626	8–53	µmol/day
Amitriptyline (therapeutic)	Serum, plasma	80–250	ng/mL	3.61	289–903	nmol/L
Ammonia (as NH_3)[b]	Plasma	15–50	µg/dL	0.714	11–35	µmol/L
Amobarbital (therapeutic)	Serum	1–5	µg/mL	4.42	4–22	µmol/L
Amoxapine (therapeutic)	Plasma	200–600	ng/mL	1	200–600	µg/L
Amylase[a,b]	Serum	27–130	U/L	0.017	0.46–2.21	µKat/L
Androstenedione,[b] male	Serum	75–205	ng/dL	0.0349	2.6–7.2	nmol/L
Androstenedione,[b] female	Serum	85–275	ng/dL	0.0349	3.0–9.6	nmol/L
Angiotensin I	Plasma	<25	pg/mL	1	<25	ng/L
Angiotensin II	Plasma	10–60	pg/mL	1	10–60	ng/L
Angiotensin-converting enzyme (ACE)[a,b]	Serum	8–52	U/L	0.017	0.14–0.88	µKat/L
Anion gap $(Na^+)-(Cl^- + HCO_3^-)$	Serum, plasma	8–16	mEq/L	1	8–16	mmol/L
Antidiuretic hormone (ADH, vasopressin) (varies with osmolality)	Plasma	1–5	pg/mL	0.926	0.9–4.6	pmol/L
Antiplasmin	Plasma	80–130	%	0.01	0.8–1.3	Fraction of 1.0
Antithrombin activity	Plasma	80–130	%	0.01	0.8–1.3	Fraction of 1.0
α₁-Antitrypsin	Serum	80–200	mg/dL	0.01	0.8–2.0	g/L
Apolipoprotein A[b]:						
Male	Serum	80–151	mg/dL	0.01	0.8–1.5	g/L
Female	Serum	80–170	mg/dL	0.01	0.8–1.7	g/L
Apolipoprotein B[b]:						
Male	Serum, plasma	50–123	mg/dL	0.01	0.5–1.2	g/L
Female	Serum, plasma	25–120	mg/dL	0.01	0.25–1.20	g/L
Arginine[b]	Plasma	0.37–2.40	mg/dL	57.4	21–138	µmol/L
Arsenic (As)	Whole blood	<23	µg/L	0.0133	<0.31	µmol/L
Arsenic (As) (chronic poisoning)	Whole blood	100–500	µg/L	0.0133	1.33–6.65	µmol/L
Arsenic (As) (acute poisoning)	Whole blood	600–9300	µg/L	0.0133	7.9–123.7	µmol/L

Continued next page—

	Specimen	Traditional Reference Interval	Traditional Units	Conversion Factor, Multiply →, ← Divide	SI Reference Interval	SI Units
Ascorbate, ascorbic acid (see vitamin C)						
Asparagine[b]	Plasma	0.40–0.91	mg/dL	75.7	30–69	µmol/L
Aspartate aminotransferase (AST, SGOT)[a,b]	Serum	20–48	U/L	0.017	0.34–0.82	µKat/L
Aspartic acid[b]	Plasma	<0.3	mg/dL	75.1	<25	µmol/L
Atrial natriuretic hormone	Plasma	20–77	pg/mL	1	20–77	ng/L
Barbiturates (see individual drugs; pentobarbital, phenobarbital, thiopental)						
Basophils (see complete blood count, white blood cell count)						
Benzodiazepines (see individual drugs; alprazolam, chlordiazepoxide, diazepam, lorazepam)						
Beryllium (toxic)	Urine	>20	µg/L	0.111	>2.22	µmol/L
Bicarbonate	Plasma	21–28	mEq/L	1	21–28	mmol/L
Bile acids (total)	Serum	0.3–2.3	µg/mL	2.448	0.73–5.63	µmol/L
Bilirubin:						
Total[b]	Serum	0.3–1.2	mg/dL	17.1	2–18	µmol/L
Direct (conjugated)	Serum	<0.2	mg/dL	17.1	<3.4	µmol/L
Biotin	Whole blood, serum	200–500	pg/mL	0.0041	0.82–2.05	nmol/L
Bismuth (therapeutic)	Whole blood	1–12	µg/L	4.785	4.8–57.4	nmol/L
Blood gases:						
P_{CO_2}	Arterial blood	35–45	mm Hg	1	35–45	mm Hg
pH	Arterial blood	7.35–7.45	—	1	7.35–7.45	—
P_{O_2}	Arterial blood	80–100	mm Hg	1	80–100	mm Hg
Blood urea nitrogen (BUN, see urea nitrogen)						
Brain natriuretic peptide (BNP)	Plasma	<100	pg/mL	1	<100	pg/mL
Bupropion (therapeutic)	Serum, plasma	25–100	ng/mL	3.62	91–362	nmol/L
C1 esterase inhibitor	Serum	12–30	mg/dL	0.01	0.12–0.30	g/L
C3 complement[b]	Serum	1200–1500	µg/mL	0.001	1.2–1.5	g/L
C4 complement[b]	Serum	350–600	µg/mL	0.001	0.35–0.60	g/L
CA125	Serum	<35	U/mL	1	<35	kU/L
CA19-9	Serum	<37	U/mL	1	<37	kU/L
CA15-3	Serum	<30	U/mL	1	<30	kU/L
CA27.29	Serum	<37.7	U/mL	1	<37.7	kU/L
Cadmium (nonsmoker)	Whole blood	0.3–1.2	µg/L	8.897	2.7–10.7	nmol/L
Caffeine (therapeutic, infants)	Serum, plasma	8–20	µg/mL	5.15	41–103	µmol/L
Calciferol (see vitamin D)						
Calcitonin	Serum, plasma	<19	pg/mL	1	<19	ng/L
Calcium, ionized	Serum	4.60–5.08	mg/dL	0.25	1.15–1.27	mmol/L
Calcium, total	Serum	8.2–10.2	mg/dL	0.25	2.05–2.55	mmol/L
Calcium, normal diet	Urine	<250	mg/24 h	0.025	<6.2	mmol/day
Carbamazepine (therapeutic)	Serum, plasma	8–12	µg/mL	4.23	34–51	µmol/L
Carbon dioxide	Serum, plasma, venous blood	22–28	mEq/L	1	22–28	mmol/L

	Specimen	Traditional Reference Interval	Traditional Units	Conversion Factor, Multiply →, ← Divide	SI Reference Interval	SI Units
Carboxyhemoglobin (carbon monoxide), as fraction of hemoglobin saturation:						
Nonsmoker	Whole blood	<2.0	%	0.01	<0.02	Fraction of 1.0
Toxic	Whole blood	>20	%	0.01	>0.2	Fraction of 1.0
β-Carotene	Serum	10–85	µg/dL	0.0186	0.2–1.6	µmol/L
Catecholamines, total (see norepinephrine)						
CEA, nonsmoker	Serum	<3	ng/mL	1	<3	µg/L
CEA, smoker	Serum	<5	ng/mL	1	<5	µg/L
Ceruloplasmin[b]	Serum	20–40	mg/dL	10	200–400	mg/L
Chloramphenicol (therapeutic)	Serum	10–25	µg/mL	3.1	31–77	µmol/L
Chlordiazepoxide (therapeutic)	Serum, plasma	0.7–1.0	µg/mL	3.34	2.3–3.3	µmol/L
Chloride	Serum, plasma	96–106	mEq/L	1	96–106	mmol/L
Chloride	CSF	118–132	mEq/L	1	118–132	mmol/L
Chlorpromazine (therapeutic, adult)	Plasma	50–300	ng/mL	3.14	157–942	nmol/L
Chlorpromazine (therapeutic, child)	Plasma	40–80	ng/mL	3.14	126–251	nmol/L
Chlorpropamide (therapeutic)	Plasma	75–250	mg/L	3.61	270–900	µmol/L
Cholesterol, high-density lipoproteins (HDL):						
Optimal	Plasma	>60	mg/dL	0.02586	>1.55	
Adequate	Plasma	40–60	mg/dL	0.02586	1.03–1.55	mmol/L
High risk for heart disease	Plasma	<40	mg/dL	0.02586	<1.03	mmol/L
Cholesterol, low-density lipoproteins (LDL)[b]:						
Optimal	Plasma	<100	mg/dL	0.02586	<2.59	mmol/L
Near optimal	Plasma	100–129	mg/dL	0.02586	2.59–3.34	mmol/L
Borderline high	Plasma	130–159	mg/dL	0.02586	3.37–4.12	mmol/L
High	Plasma	160–189	mg/dL	0.02586	4.15–4.90	mmol/L
Very high	Plasma	>190	mg/dL	0.02586	>4.90	mmol/L
Cholesterol total, adult:						
Desirable	Serum	<200	mg/dL	0.02586	<5.17	mmol/L
Borderline high	Serum	200–239	mg/dL	0.02586	5.17–6.18	mmol/L
High	Serum	>240	mg/dL	0.02586	>6.21	mmol/L
Cholesterol total, children:						
Desirable	Serum	<170	mg/dL	0.02586	4.4	mmol/L
Borderline high	Serum	170–199	mg/dL	0.02586	4.40–5.15	mmol/L
High	Serum	>200	mg/dL	0.02586	>5.18	mmol/L
Chromium	Whole blood	0.7–28.0	µg/L	19.2	13.4–538.6	nmol/L
Citrate	Serum	1.2–3.0	mg/dL	52.05	60–160	µmol/L
Citrulline[b]	Plasma	0.4–2.4	mg/dL	57.1	20–135	µmol/L
Clonazepam (therapeutic)	Serum	15–60	ng/mL	3.17	48–190	nmol/L

Continued next page—

	Specimen	Traditional Reference Interval	Traditional Units	Conversion Factor, Multiply →, ← Divide	SI Reference Interval	SI Units
Coagulation factor I (fibrinogen)	Plasma	150–400	mg/dL	0.01	1.5–4.0	g/L
Coagulation factor II (prothrombin)	Plasma	60–140	%	0.01	0.60–1.40	Fraction of 1.0
Coagulation factor V	Plasma	60–140	%	0.01	0.60–1.40	Fraction of 1.0
Coagulation factor VII	Plasma	60–140	%	0.01	0.60–1.40	Fraction of 1.0
Coagulation factor VIII	Plasma	50–200	%	0.01	0.50–2.00	Fraction of 1.0
Coagulation factor IX	Plasma	60–140	%	0.01	0.60–1.40	Fraction of 1.0
Coagulation factor X	Plasma	60–140	%	0.01	0.60–1.40	Fraction of 1.0
Coagulation factor XI	Plasma	60–140	%	0.01	0.60–1.40	Fraction of 1.0
Coagulation factor XII	Plasma	60–140	%	0.01	0.60–1.40	Fraction of 1.0
Cobalt	Serum	<1.0	µg/L	16.97	<17	nmol/L
Codeine (therapeutic)	Serum	10–100	ng/mL	3.34	33–334	nmol/L
Complete blood count (CBC):						
Hematocrit[b]:						
Male	Whole blood	41–50	%	0.01	0.41–0.50	Fraction of 1.0
Female	Whole blood	35–45	%	0.01	0.35–0.45	Fraction of 1.0
Hemoglobin (mass concentration)[b]:						
Male	Whole blood	13.5–17.5	g/dL	10	135–175	g/L
Female	Whole blood	12.0–15.5	g/dL	10	120–155	g/L
Hemoglobin (substance concentration, Hb [Fe]):						
Male	Whole blood	13.6–17.2	g/dL	0.6206	8.44–10.65	mmol/L
Female	Whole blood	12.0–15.0	g/dL	0.6206	7.45–9.30	mmol/L
Mean corpuscular hemoglobin (MCH), mass concentration[b]	Whole blood	27–33	pg/cell	1	27–33	pg/cell
MCH, substance concentration, Hb [Fe]	Whole blood	27–33	pg/cell	0.06206	1.70–2.05	fmol
Mean corpuscular hemoglobin concentration (MCHC), mass concentration	Whole blood	33–37	g Hb/dL	10	330–370	g Hb/L
MCHC, substance concentration, Hb [Fe]	Whole blood	33–37	g Hb/dL	0.6206	20–23	mmol/L
Mean cell volume (MCV)[b]	Whole blood	80–100	µm^3	1	80–100	fL
Platelet count	Whole blood	150–450	$10^3 \, \mu L^{-1}$	1	150–450	$10^9 \, L^{-1}$
Red blood cell count:						
Female	Whole blood	3.9–5.5	$10^6 \, \mu L^{-1}$	1	3.9–5.5	$10^{12} \, L^{-1}$
Male	Whole blood	4.6–6.0	$10^6 \, \mu L^{-1}$	1	4.6–6.0	$10^{12} \, L^{-1}$
Reticulocyte count[b]	Whole blood	25–75	$10^3 \, \mu L^{-1}$	1	25–75	$10^9 \, L^{-1}$
Reticulocyte count[b] (fraction)	Whole blood	0.5–1.5	% of RBCs	0.01	0.005–0.015	Fraction of RBCs
White blood cell count[b]	Whole blood	4.5–11.0	$10^3 \, \mu L^{-1}$	1	4.5–11.0	$10^9 \, L^{-1}$

	Specimen	Traditional Reference Interval	Traditional Units	Conversion Factor, Multiply →, ← Divide	SI Reference Interval	SI Units
Differential count[b] (absolute):						
Neutrophils	Whole blood	1800–7800	μL^{-1}	1	1.8–7.8	$10^9 L^{-1}$
Bands	Whole blood	0–700	μL^{-1}	1	0.00–0.70	$10^9 L^{-1}$
Lymphocytes	Whole blood	1000–4800	μL^{-1}	1	1.0–4.8	$10^9 L^{-1}$
Monocytes	Whole blood	0–800	μL^{-1}	1	0.00–0.80	$10^9 L^{-1}$
Eosinophils	Whole blood	0–450	μL^{-1}	1	0.00–0.45	$10^9 L^{-1}$
Basophils	Whole blood	0–200	μL^{-1}	1	0.00–0.20	$10^9 L^{-1}$
Differential count[b] (number fraction):						
Neutrophils	Whole blood	56	%	0.01	0.56	Fraction of 1.0
Bands	Whole blood	3	%	0.01	0.03	Fraction of 1.0
Lymphocytes	Whole blood	34	%	0.01	0.34	Fraction of 1.0
Monocytes	Whole blood	4	%	0.01	0.04	Fraction of 1.0
Eosinophils	Whole blood	2.7	%	0.01	0.027	Fraction of 1.0
Basophils	Whole blood	0.3	%	0.01	0.003	Fraction of 1.0
Copper[b]	Serum	70–140	$\mu g/dL$	0.1574	11.0–22.0	$\mu mol/L$
Coproporphyrin	Urine	<200	$\mu g/24\ h$	1.527	<300	nmol/day
Corticotropin[b] (08:00)	Plasma	<120	pg/mL	0.22	<26	pmol/L
Cortisol, total[b]:						
Time of day:						
8:00	Plasma	5–25	$\mu g/dL$	27.6	138–690	nmol/L
16:00	Plasma	3–16	$\mu g/dL$	27.6	83–442	nmol/L
20:00	Plasma	<50% of 08:00	$\mu g/dL$	1	<50% of 08:00	nmol/L
Cortisol, free[b]	Urine	30–100	$\mu g/24\ h$	2.76	80–280	nmol/day
Cotinine (smoker)	Plasma	16–145	ng/mL	5.68	91–823	nmol/L
C-peptide	Serum	0.5–3.5	ng/mL	0.333	0.17–1.17	nmol/L
Creatine, male	Serum	0.2–0.7	mg/dL	76.3	15.3–53.3	$\mu mol/L$
Creatine, female	Serum	0.3–0.9	mg/dL	76.3	22.9–68.6	$\mu mol/L$
Creatine kinase (CK)[a]	Serum	50–200	U/L	0.017	0.85–3.40	$\mu Kat/L$
CK-MB fraction	Serum	<6	%	0.01	<0.06	Fraction of 1.0
Creatinine[b]	Serum, plasma	0.6–1.2	mg/dL	88.4	53–106	$\mu mol/L$
Creatinine	Urine	1–2	g/24 h	8.84	8.8–17.7	mmol/day
Creatinine clearance, glomerular filtration rate	Serum, urine	75–125	$mL/min/1.73\ m^2$	0.00963	0.72–1.2	$mL/s/m^2$
C-telopeptide:						
Men	Serum, plasma	60–700	pg/mL	1	60–700	pg/mL
Premenopausal women	Serum, plasma	40–465	pg/mL	1	40–465	pg/mL
Cyanide (toxic)	Whole blood	>1.0	$\mu g/mL$	38.4	>38.4	$\mu mol/L$

Continued next page—

	Specimen	Traditional Reference Interval	Traditional Units	Conversion Factor, Multiply →, ← Divide	SI Reference Interval	SI Units
Cyanocobalamin (see vitamin B₁₂)						
Cyclic adenosine monophosphate (cAMP)	Plasma	4.6–8.6	ng/mL	3.04	14–26	nmol/L
Cyclosporine (toxic)	Whole blood	>400	ng/mL	0.832	>333	nmol/L
Cystine[b]	Plasma	0.40–1.40	mg/dL	83.3	33–117	μmol/L
D-dimer[b]	Plasma	Negative (<500)	ng/mL	1	Negative (<500)	ng/mL
Dehydroepiandrosterone (DHEA) (unconjugated, male)[b]	Plasma, serum	180–1250	ng/dL	0.0347	6.2–43.3	nmol/L
Dehydroepiandrosterone sulfate (DHEA-S) (male)[b]	Plasma, serum	10–619	μg/dL	0.027	0.3–16.7	μmol/L
Desipramine (therapeutic)	Plasma, serum	50–200	ng/mL	3.75	170–700	nmol/L
Diazepam (therapeutic)	Plasma, serum	100–1000	ng/mL	0.00351	0.35–3.51	μmol/L
Digoxin (therapeutic)	Plasma	0.5–2.0	ng/mL	1.281	0.6–2.6	nmol/L
Disopyramide (therapeutic)	Plasma, serum	2.8–7.0	mg/L	2.95	8–21	μmol/L
Doxepin (therapeutic)	Plasma, serum	150–250	ng/mL	3.58	540–890	nmol/L
Electrolytes:						
Chloride	Serum, plasma	96–106	mEq/L	1	96–106	mmol/L
Carbon dioxide (CO₂)	Serum, plasma, venous blood	22–28	mEq/L	1	22–28	mmol/L
Potassium	Plasma	3.5–5.0	mEq/L	1	3.5–5.0	mmol/L
Sodium[b]	Plasma	136–142	mEq/L	1	136–142	mmol/L
Eosinophils (see complete blood count, white blood cell count)						
Epinephrine (supine)	Plasma	<50	pg/mL	5.46	<273	pmol/L
Epinephrine[b]	Urine	<20	μg/24 h	5.46	<109	nmol/day
Erythrocyte count (see complete blood count, red blood cell count)						
Erythrocyte sedimentation rate (ESR)[b]	Whole blood	0–20	mm/h	1	0–20	mm/h
Erythropoietin	Serum	5–36	mU/mL	1	5–36	IU/L
Estradiol (E2, unconjugated),[b] female:						
Follicular phase	Serum	20–350	pg/mL	3.69	73–1285	pmol/L
Midcycle peak	Serum	150–750	pg/mL	3.69	551–2753	pmol/L
Luteal phase	Serum	30–450	pg/mL	3.69	110–1652	pmol/L
Postmenopausal	Serum	<59	pg/mL	3.69	<218	pmol/L
Estradiol (unconjugated),[b] male	Serum	<20	pg/mL	3.67	<184	pmol/L
Estriol (E3, unconjugated), males and nonpregnant females, varies with length of gestation	Serum	<2	ng/mL	3.47	<6.9	nmol/L
Estrogens (total),[b] female:						
Follicular phase	Serum	60–200	pg/mL	1	60–200	ng/L
Luteal phase	Serum	160–400	pg/mL	1	160–400	ng/L

	Specimen	Traditional Reference Interval	Traditional Units	Conversion Factor, Multiply →, ← Divide	SI Reference Interval	SI Units
Postmenopausal	Serum	<130	pg/mL	1	<130	ng/L
Estrogens (total),[b] male	Serum	20–80	pg/mL	1	20–80	ng/L
Estrone (E1),[b] female:						
Follicular phase	Plasma, serum	100–250	pg/mL	3.69	370–925	pmol/L
Luteal phase	Plasma, serum	15–200	pg/mL	3.69	55–740	pmol/L
Postmenopausal	Plasma, serum	15–55	pg/mL	3.69	55–204	pmol/L
Estrone (E1),[b] male	Plasma, serum	15–65	pg/mL	3.69	55–240	pmol/L
Ethanol (ethyl alcohol) (legal intoxication—2 levels listed)	Serum, whole blood	>80 / >100	mg/dL	0.2171	>17.4 / 21.7	mmol/L
Ethosuximide (therapeutic)	Plasma, serum	40–100	µg/mL	7.08	283–708	µmol/L
Ethylene glycol (toxic)	Plasma, serum	>30	mg/dL	0.1611	>5	mmol/L
Everolimus (therapeutic)	Whole blood	3–15	ng/mL	1.04	5–16	nmol/L
Fatty acids (nonesterified)	Plasma	8–25	mg/dL	0.0354	0.28–0.89	mmol/L
Fecal fat (as stearic acid)	Stool	2.0–6.0	g/day	1	2–6	g/day
Felbamate (therapeutic)	Serum, plasma	30–60	µg/mL	4.2	126–252	µmol/L
Ferritin[b]	Plasma	15–200	ng/mL	1	15–200	µg/L
α-Fetoprotein[b]	Serum	<10	ng/mL	1	<10	µg/L
Fibrinogen	Plasma	150–400	mg/dL	0.01	1.5–4.0	g/L
Fibrin breakdown products (fibrin split products)	Serum	<10	µg/mL	1	<10	mg/L
Folate (folic acid)	Red blood cells	166–640	ng/mL	2.266	376–1450	nmol/L
Folate (folic acid)	Serum	5–25	ng/mL	2.266	11–57	nmol/L
Follicle-stimulating hormone (FSH),[b] female:						
Follicular phase	Serum	1.37–9.9	mIU/mL	1	1.3–9.9	IU/L
Ovulatory phase	Serum	6.17–17.2	mIU/mL	1	6.1–17.2	IU/L
Luteal phase	Serum	1.09–9.2	mIU/mL	1	1.0–9.2	IU/L
Postmenopausal	Serum	19.3–100.6	mIU/mL	1	19.3–100.6	IU/L
FSH[b] male	Serum	1.42–15.4	mIU/mL	1	1.4–15.4	IU/L
FSH[b] female	Urine	2–15	IU/24 h	1	2–15	IU/day
FSH[b] male	Urine	3–12	IU/24 h	1	3–11	IU/day
Fructosamine[b]	Serum	1.5–2.7	mmol/L	1	1.5–2.7	mmol/L
Gabapentin (therapeutic)	Serum, plasma	2–20	µg/mL	5.84	12–117	µmol/L
Gastrin (fasting)	Serum	<100	pg/mL	1	<100	ng/L
Gentamicin (therapeutic)	Serum	6–10	µg/mL	2.1	12–21	µmol/L
Glucagon[b]	Plasma	20–100	pg/mL	1	20–100	ng/L
Glucose[b]	Serum, plasma	70–110	mg/dL	0.05551	3.9–6.1	mmol/L
Glucose	CSF	50–80	mg/dL	0.05551	2.8–4.4	mmol/L
Glucose-6-phosphate dehydrogenase	Red blood cells	10–14	U/g of Hb	0.0645	0.65–0.90	U/mol of Hb

Continued next page—

	Specimen	Traditional Reference Interval	Traditional Units	Conversion Factor, Multiply →, ← Divide	SI Reference Interval	SI Units
Glutamic acid[b]	Plasma	0.2–2.8	mg/dL	67.97	15–190	μmol/L
Glutamine	Plasma	6.1–10.2	mg/dL	68.42	420–700	μmol/L
γ-Glutamyltransferase (GGT; γ-glutamyl transpeptidase)[b]:						
Female	Serum	<30	U/L	0.017	0.51	μKat/L
Male	Serum	<50	U/L	0.017	<0.85	μKat/L
Glycerol (free)[b]	Serum	<1.5	mg/dL	0.1086	<0.16	mmol/L
Glycine[b]	Plasma	0.9–4.2	mg/dL	133.3	120–560	μmol/L
Glycated hemoglobin (hemoglobin A1, A1c):						
Whole blood	Whole blood	4–5.6	% of total Hb	1	4–5.6	Fraction of total Hb
Gold (therapeutic)	Serum	100–200	μg/dL	0.05077	5.1–10.2	μmol/L
Growth hormone, adult (GH, somatotropin)[b]	Plasma, serum	<10	ng/mL	1	<10	μg/L
Haloperidol (therapeutic)	Serum, plasma	5–20	ng/mL	2.6	13–52	nmol/L
Haptoglobin[b]	Serum	40–180	mg/dL	0.01	0.4–1.8	g/L
Hematocrit (see complete blood count)						
Hemoglobin (see complete blood count)						
Hemoglobin A1c (see glycated hemoglobin)						
Hemoglobin A2[b]	Whole blood	2.0–3.5	% total Hb		2.0–3.5	Fraction of 1.0
Hemoglobin F[b] (fetal hemoglobin in adult)	Whole blood	<2	%	0.01	<2	Fraction of 1.0
Histidine[b]	Plasma	0.5–1.7	mg/dL	64.5	32–110	μmol/L
Homocysteine (total)	Plasma, serum	4–12	μmol/L	1	4–12	μmol/L
Homovanillic acid[b]	Urine	<8	mg/24 h	5.489	<45	μmol/day
Human chorionic gonadotropin (hCG) (nonpregnant adult female)	Serum	<3	mIU/mL	1	<3	IU/L
β-Hydroxybutyric acid	Serum	0.21–2.81	mg/dL	96.05	20–270	μmol/L
5-Hydroxyindoleacetic acid (5-HIAA)	Urine	<25	mg/24 h	5.23	<131	μmol/day
17α-Hydroxyprogesterone,[b] female:						
Follicular phase	Serum	15–70	ng/dL	0.03	0.4–2.1	nmol/L
Luteal phase	Serum	35–290	ng/dL	0.03	1.0–8.7	nmol/L
Postmenopausal	Serum	<70	ng/dL	0.03	<2.1	nmol/L
17α-Hydroxyprogesterone,[b] male	Serum	27–199	ng/dL	0.03	0.8–6.0	nmol/L
Hydroxyproline	Plasma	<0.55	mg/dL	76.3	<42	μmol/L
5-Hydroxytryptamine (see serotonin)						
Ibuprofen (therapeutic)	Serum, plasma	10–50	μg/mL	4.85	49–243	μmol/L
Imipramine (therapeutic)	Serum, plasma	150–250	ng/mL	3.57	536–893	nmol/L
Immunoglobulin A (IgA)[b]	Serum	50–350	mg/dL	0.01	0.5–3.5	g/L
Immunoglobulin D (IgD)	Serum	0.5–3.0	mg/dL	10	5–30	mg/L

	Specimen	Traditional Reference Interval	Traditional Units	Conversion Factor, Multiply →, ← Divide	SI Reference Interval	SI Units
Immunoglobulin E (IgE)	Serum	10–179	IU/mL	2.4	24–430	µg/L
Immunoglobulin G (IgG)[b]	Serum	600–1560	mg/dL	0.01	6.0–15.6	g/L
Immunoglobulin M (IgM)[b]	Serum	54–222	mg/dL	0.01	0.5–2.2	g/L
Insulin	Plasma	5–20	µU/mL	6.945	34.7–138.9	pmol/L
Inhibin A:						
Males	Serum	1.0–3.6	pg/mL	1	1.0–3.6	ng/L
Female, early follicular	Serum	5.5–28.2	pg/mL	1	5.5–28.2	ng/L
Female, late follicular	Serum	19.5–102.3	pg/mL	1	19.5–102.3	ng/L
Female, midcycle	Serum	49.9–155.5	pg/mL	1	49.9–155.5	ng/L
Female, midluteal	Serum	13.2–159.6	pg/mL	1	13.2–159.6	ng/L
Female, postmenopausal	Serum	1.0–3.9	pg/mL	1	1.0–3.9	ng/L
Insulin C-peptide (see C-peptide)						
Insulin-like growth factor[b]	Serum	130–450	ng/mL	1	130–450	µg/L
Ionized calcium (see calcium)						
Iron (total)[b]	Serum	60–150	µg/dL	0.179	10.7–26.9	µmol/L
Iron-binding capacity	Serum	250–400	µg/dL	0.179	44.8–71.6	µmol/L
Isoleucine[b]	Plasma	0.5–1.3	mg/dL	76.24	40–100	µmol/L
Isoniazid (therapeutic)	Plasma or serum	1–7	µg/mL	7.29	7–51	µmol/L
Isopropanol (toxic)	Plasma, serum	>400	mg/L	0.0166	>6.64	mmol/L
Lactate (lactic acid)	Arterial blood	3–11.3	mg/dL	0.111	0.3–1.3	mmol/L
Lactate (lactic acid)	Venous blood	4.5–19.8	mg/dL	0.111	0.5–2.2	mmol/L
Lactate dehydrogenase (LDH, LD)	Serum	50–200	U/L	1	50–200	U/L
Lamotrigine (therapeutic)	Serum, plasma	2.5–15	µg/dL	3.91	10–59	µmol/L
Lead (toxic)	Whole blood	>5	µg/dL	0.0483	>0.24	µmol/L
Leucine[b]	Plasma	1.0–2.3	mg/dL	76.3	75–175	µmol/L
Leukocyte count (see complete blood count, white blood cell count)						
Levetiracetam (therapeutic)	Serum, plasma	12–46	µg/mL	5.88	71–270	µmol/L
Lidocaine (therapeutic)	Serum, plasma	1.5–6.0	mg/mL	4.27	6.4–25.6	µmol/L
Lipase[a]	Serum	0–160	U/L	0.017	0–2.72	µKat/L
Lipoprotein(a) (Lp(a))	Serum, plasma	10–30	mg/dL	0.01	0.1–0.3	g/L
Lithium (therapeutic)	Serum, plasma	0.6–1.2	mEq/L	1	0.6–1.2	mmol/L
Lorazepam (therapeutic)	Serum, plasma	50–240	ng/mL	3.11	156–746	nmol/L
Luteinizing hormone (LH),[b] female:						
Follicular phase	Serum	2.0–15.0	mIU/L	1	2.0–15.0	IU/L
Ovulatory peak	Serum	22.0–105.0	mIU/L	1	22.0–105.0	IU/L
Luteal phase	Serum	0.6–19.0	mIU/L	1	0.6–19.0	IU/L
Postmenopausal	Serum	16.0–64.0	mIU/L	1	16.0–64.0	IU/L
Luteinizing hormone (LH),[b] male	Serum	2.0–12.0	mIU/L	1	2.0–12.0	IU/L

Continued next page—

	Specimen	Traditional Reference Interval	Traditional Units	Conversion Factor, Multiply →, ← Divide	SI Reference Interval	SI Units
Lymphocytes (see complete blood count, white blood cell count)						
Lysine[b]	Plasma	1.2–3.5	mg/dL	68.5	80–240	µmol/L
Lysozyme (muramidase)	Serum	4–13	mg/L	1	4–13	mg/L
Magnesium[b]	Serum	1.5–2.5	mg/dL	0.4114	0.62–1.03	mmol/L
Manganese	Whole blood	10–12	µg/L	18.2	182–218	nmol/L
Maprotiline (therapeutic)	Plasma, serum	200–600	ng/mL	1	200–600	µg/L
MCH (see complete blood count)						
MCHC (see complete blood count)						
Meperidine (therapeutic)	Serum, plasma	0.4–0.7	µg/mL	4.04	1.6–2.8	µmol/L
Mercury	Whole blood	0.6–59.0	µg/L	4.99	3.0–294.4	nmol/L
Metanephrines (total)[b]	Urine	<1.0	mg/24 h	5.07	<5	µmol/day
Methadone (therapeutic)	Serum, plasma	100–400	ng/mL	0.00323	0.32–1.29	µmol/L
Methanol (toxic)	Whole blood, serum	>1.5	mg/L	0.0312	>0.05	mmol/L
Methemoglobin	Whole blood	<0.24	g/dL	155	<37.2	µmol/L
Methemoglobin	Whole blood	<1.0	% of total Hb	0.01	<0.01	Fraction of total Hb
Methionine[b]	Plasma	0.1–0.6	mg/dL	67.1	6–40	µmol/L
Methsuximide (therapeutic)	Serum, plasma	10–40	µg/mL	5.29	53–212	µmol/L
Methyldopa (therapeutic)	Serum, plasma	1–5	µg/mL	4.73	5–24	µmol/L
Metoprolol (therapeutic)	Serum, plasma	75–200	ng/mL	3.74	281–748	nmol/L
Mexthotrexate:						
Toxic 24 h after dose	Serum, plasma	≥10	µmol/L	1	≥10	µmol/L
Toxic 48 h after dose	Serum, plasma	≥1	µmol/L	1	≥1	µmol/L
Toxic 72 h after dose	Serum, plasma	≥0.1	µmol/L	1	≥0.1	µmol/L
β_2-Microglobulin	Serum	<2	µg/mL	85	<170	nmol/L
Monocytes (see complete blood count, white blood cell count)						
Morphine (therapeutic)	Serum, plasma	10–80	ng/mL	3.5	35–280	nmol/L
Muramidase (see lysozyme)						
Mycophenolic acid (therapeutic)	Serum, plasma	1.3–3.5	µg/mL	3.12	4–11	µmol/L
Naproxen (therapeutic)	Plasma, serum	>50	µg/mL	4.34	>217	µmol/L
Neutrophils (see complete blood count, white blood cell count)						
Niacin (Vitamin B_3, nicotinic acid)	Plasma, serum	0.50–8.45	ug/mL	7.3	3.65–61.69	µmol/day
Nickel	Whole blood	1.0–28.0	µg/L	17	17–476	nmol/L
Nicotine (smoker)	Plasma	0.01–0.05	mg/L	6.16	0.062–0.308	µmol/L
Norepinephrine[b]	Plasma	110–410	pg/mL	5.91	650–2423	nmol/L
Norepinephrine[b]	Urine	15–80	µg/24 h	5.91	89–473	nmol/day
Nortriptyline (therapeutic)	Serum, plasma	50–150	ng/mL	3.8	190–570	nmol/L

	Specimen	Traditional Reference Interval	Traditional Units	Conversion Factor, Multiply →, ← Divide	SI Reference Interval	SI Units
N-telopeptide (BCE, bone collagen equivalents):						
Men	Serum	5.4–24.2	nmol BCE/L	1	5.4–24.2	nmol BCE/L
Premenopausal women	Serum	6.2–19.0	nmol BCE/L	1	6.2–19.0	nmol BCE/L
Ornithine[b]	Plasma	0.4–1.4	mg/dL	75.8	30–106	μmol/L
Osmolality[b]	Serum	275–295	mOsm/kg H$_2$O	1	275–295	mmol/kg H$_2$O
Osmolality	Urine	250–900	mOsm/kg H$_2$O	1	250–900	mmol/kg H$_2$O
Osteocalcin[b]	Serum	3.0–13.0	ng/mL	1	3.0–13.0	μg/L
Oxalate	Serum	1.0–2.4	mg/L	11.4	11–27	μmol/L
Oxazepam (therapeutic)	Serum, plasma	0.2–1.4	μg/mL	3.49	0.7–54.9	μmol/L
Oxycodone (therapeutic)	Plasma, serum	10–100	ng/mL	3.17	32–317	nmol/L
Oxygen, partial pressure (Po$_2$)	Arterial blood	80–100	mm Hg	1	80–100	mm Hg
Pantothenic acid (see vitamin B$_5$)						
Parathyroid hormone:						
Intact[b]	Serum	10–50	pg/mL	1	10–50	ng/L
N-terminal specific[b]	Serum	8–24	pg/mL	1	8–24	ng/L
C-terminal (mid-molecule)	Serum	0–340	pg/mL	1	0–340	ng/L
Pentobarbital (therapeutic)	Serum, plasma	1–5	μg/mL	4.42	4.0–22	μmol/L
Pepsinogen I[b]	Serum	28–100	ng/mL	1	28–100	μg/L
pH (see blood gases)						
Phenobarbital (therapeutic)	Serum, plasma	15–40	μg/mL	4.31	65–172	μmol/L
Phenylalanine[b]	Plasma	0.6–1.5	mg/dL	60.5	35–90	μmol/L
Phenytoin (therapeutic)	Serum, plasma	10–20	μg/mL	3.96	40–79	μmol/L
Phosphatase, tartrate-resistant acid	Serum	1.5–4.5	U/L	0.017	0.03–0.08	μkat/L
Phosphorus (inorganic)[b]	Serum	2.3–4.7	mg/dL	0.3229	0.74–1.52	mmol/L
Phosphorus (inorganic)[b]	Urine	0.4–1.3	g/24 h	32.29	12.9–42.0	mmol/day
Plasminogen	Plasma	80–120	%	0.01	0.80–1.20	Fraction of 1.0
Plasminogen activator inhibitor activity	Plasma	3–56	mIU/mL	1	3–56	IU/L
Platelet count (see complete blood count, platelet count)						
Porphobilinogen deaminase	Red blood cells	>7.0	nmol/s/L	1	>7.0	nmol/(s L)
Potassium	Plasma	3.5–5.0	mEq/L	1	3.5–5.0	mmol/L
Prealbumin—transthyretin	Serum, plasma	18–45	mg/dL	0.01	0.18–0.45	g/L
Pregnanediol,[b] female:						
Follicular phase	Urine	<2.6	mg/24 h	3.12	<8	μmol/day
Luteal phase	Urine	2.3–10.6	mg/24 h	3.12	8–33	μmol/day
Pregnanediol,[b] male	Urine	0–1.9	mg/24 h	3.12	0–5.9	μmol/day
Pregnanetriol[b]	Urine	<2.5	mg/24 h	2.97	<7.5	μmol/day

Continued next page—

	Specimen	Traditional Reference Interval	Traditional Units	Conversion Factor, Multiply →, ← Divide	SI Reference Interval	SI Units
Primidone (therapeutic)	Serum, plasma	12 May	μg/mL	4.58	23–55	μmol/L
Procainamide (therapeutic)	Serum, plasma	10 Apr	μg/mL	4.23	17–42	μmol/L
Progesterone,[b] female:						
Follicular phase	Serum	0.1–0.7	ng/mL	3.18	0.5–2.2	nmol/L
Luteal phase	Serum	2.0–25.0	ng/mL	3.18	6.4–79.5	nmol/L
Progesterone,[b] male	Serum	0.13–0.97	ng/mL	3.18	0.4–3.1	nmol/L
Prolactin (nonlactating subject)	Serum	1–25	ng/mL	1	1–25	μg/L
Proline[b]	Plasma	1.2–3.9	mg/dL	86.9	104–340	μmol/L
Propoxyphene (therapeutic)	Serum	0.1–0.4	μg/mL	2.946	0.3–1.2	μmol/L
Propanolol (therapeutic)	Serum, plasma	50–100	ng/mL	3.86	190–386	nmol/L
Protein (total)[b]	Serum	6.0–8.0	g/dL	10	60–80	g/L
Protein C activity	Plasma	70–140	%	0.01	0.70–1.40	Fraction of 1.0
Protein electrophoresis (serum protein electrophoresis [SPEP]), fraction of total protein:						
Albumin	Serum	52–65	%	0.01	0.52–0.65	Fraction of 1.0
α_1-Globulin	Serum	2.5–5.0	%	0.01	0.025–0.05	Fraction of 1.0
α_2-Globulin	Serum	7.0–13.0	%	0.01	0.07–0.13	Fraction of 1.0
β-Globulin	Serum	8.0–14.0	%	0.01	0.08–0.14	Fraction of 1.0
γ-Globulin	Serum	12.0–22.0	%	0.01	0.12–0.22	Fraction of 1.0
Protein electrophoresis (SPEP), concentration:						
Albumin	Serum	3.2–5.6	g/dL	10	32–56	g/L
α_1-Globulin	Serum	0.1–0.4	g/dL	10	1–10	g/L
α_2-Globulin	Serum	0.4–1.2	g/dL	10	4–12	g/L
β-Globulin	Serum	0.5–1.1	g/dL	10	5–11	g/L
γ-Globulin	Serum	0.5–1.6	g/dL	10	5–16	g/L
Protein S activity	Plasma	70–140	%	0.01	0.70–1.40	Fraction of 1.0
Protein S free antigen	Plasma	80–160	%	0.01	0.80–1.60	Fraction of 1.0
Prothrombin time (PT)	Plasma	10–13	seconds	1	10–13	seconds
Protoporphyrin	Red blood cells	15–50	μg/dL	0.0177	0.27–0.89	μmol/L
Prostate-specific antigen (PSA)	Serum	0–4.0	ng/mL	1	0–4.0	μg/L
Pyridinium cross-links (deoxypyridinoline):						
Male	Urine	10.3–20	nmol/mmol creatinine	1	10.3–20	nmol/mmol creatinine
Premenopausal female	Urine	15.3–33.6	nmol/mmol creatinine	1	15.3–33.6	nmol/mmol creatinine
Pyridoxine (see vitamin B$_6$)						
Pyruvate (as pyruvic acid)	Whole blood	0.3–0.9	mg/dL	113.6	34–102	μmol/L
Quinidine (therapeutic)	Serum, plasma	2.0–5.0	μg/mL	3.08	6.2–15.4	μmol/L

	Specimen	Traditional Reference Interval	Traditional Units	Conversion Factor, Multiply →, ← Divide	SI Reference Interval	SI Units
Red blood cell count (see complete blood count)						
Red cell folate (see folate)						
Renin (normal-sodium diet)[b]	Plasma	1.1–4.1	ng/mL/h	1	1.1–4.1	ng/(mL h)
Reticulocyte count[b]	Whole blood	25–75	$10^3\,\mu L^{-1}$	1	25–75	$10^9\,L^{-1}$
Reticulocyte count[b] (fraction)	Whole blood	0.5–1.5	% of RBCs	0.01	0.005–0.015	Fraction of RBCs
Retinol (see vitamin A)						
Rheumatoid factor	Serum	<30	IU/mL	1	<30	kIU/L
Riboflavin (see vitamin B_2)						
Salicylates (therapeutic)	Serum, plasma	15–30	mg/dL	0.0724	1.08–2.17	mmol/L
Sedimentation rate (see erythrocyte sedimentation rate)						
Selenium	Whole blood	58–234	µg/L	0.0127	0.74–2.97	µmol/L
Serine[b]	Plasma	0.7–2.0	mg/dL	95.2	65–193	µmol/L
Serotonin (5-hydroxytryptamine)	Whole blood	50–200	ng/mL	0.00568	0.28–1.14	µmol/L
Sertraline (therapeutic)	Serum or plasma	10–50	ng/mL	3.27	33–164	nmol/L
SPEP (see protein electrophoresis)						
Sex hormone-binding globulin[b]	Serum	0.5–1.5	µg/dL	34.7	17.4–52.1	nmol/L
Sirolimus (therapeutic)	Whole blood	4–20	ng/mL	1.1	4–22	nmol/L
Sodium[b]	Plasma	136–142	mEq/L	1	136–142	mmol/L
Somatostatin	Plasma	<25	pg/mL	1	<25	ng/L
Somatomedin C (see insulin-like growth factor)						
Strychnine (toxic)	Whole blood	>0.5	mg/L	2.99	>1.5	µmol/L
Substance P	Plasma	<240	pg/mL	1	<240	ng/L
Sulfhemoglobin	Whole blood	<1.0	% of total Hb	0.01	<0.010	Fraction of total Hb
Tacrolimus (therapeutic)	Whole blood	3–20	ng/mL	1.24	4–25	nmol/L
Taurine[b]	Plasma	0.3–2.1	mg/dL	80	24–168	µmol/L
Testosterone,[b] male	Plasma, serum	300–1200	ng/dL	0.0347	10.4–41.6	nmol/L
Testosterone,[b] female	Plasma, serum	<85	ng/dL	0.0347	2.95	nmol/L
Theophylline (therapeutic)	Plasma, serum	10–20	µg/mL	5.55	56–111	µmol/L
Thiamine (see vitamin B_1)						
Thiocyanate (nonsmoker)	Plasma, serum	1–4	mg/L	17.2	17–69	µmol/L
Thiopental (therapeutic)	Plasma, serum	1–5	µg/mL	4.13	4–21	µmol/L
Thioridazine (therapeutic)	Plasma, serum	1.0–1.5	µg/mL	2.7	2.7–4.1	µmol/L
Thrombin time	Plasma	16–24	seconds	1	16–24	seconds
Threonine[b]	Plasma	0.9–2.5	mg/dL	84	75–210	µmol/L

Continued next page—

	Specimen	Traditional Reference Interval	Traditional Units	Conversion Factor, Multiply →, ← Divide	SI Reference Interval	SI Units
Thyroglobulin[b]	Serum	3–42	ng/mL	1	3–42	µg/L
Thyrotropin (thyroid-stimulating hormone, TSH)[b]	Serum	0.5–5.0	µIU/mL	1	0.5–5.0	mU/L
Thyroxine, free (FT$_4$)[b]	Serum	0.9–2.3	ng/dL	12.87	12–30	pmol/L
Thyroxine, total (T$_4$)[b]	Serum	5.5–12.5	µg/dL	12.87	71–160	nmol/L
Thyroxine-binding globulin (TBG),[b] as T$_4$ binding capacity	Serum	10–26	µg/dL	12.9	129–335	nmol/L
Tissue plasminogen activator	Plasma	<0.04	IU/mL	1000	<40	IU/L
Tobramycin (therapeutic)	Plasma, serum	5–10	µg/mL	2.14	10–21	µmol/L
Tocainide (therapeutic)	Plasma, serum	4–10	µg/mL	5.2	21–52	µmol/L
α-Tocopherol (see vitamin E)						
Topiramate (therapeutic)	Serum, plasma	5–20	µg/mL	2.95	15–59	µmol/L
Transferrin (siderophilin)[b]	Serum	200–380	mg/dL	0.01	2.0–3.8	g/L
Triglycerides[b]	Plasma, serum	10–190	mg/dL	0.01129	0.11–2.15	mmol/L
Triiodothyronine, free (FT$_3$)[b]	Serum	260–480	pg/dL	0.0154	4.0–7.4	pmol/L
Triiodothyronine, resin uptake[b]	Serum	25–35	%	0.01	0.25–0.35	Fraction of 1.0
Triiodothyronine, total (T$_3$)[b]	Serum	70–200	ng/dL	0.0154	1.08–3.14	nmol/L
Troponin I (cardiac)	Serum	0–0.4	ng/mL	1	0–0.4	µg/L
Troponin T (cardiac)	Serum	0–0.1	ng/mL	1	0–0.1	µg/L
Tryptophan[b]	Plasma	0.5–1.5	mg/dL	48.97	25–73	µmol/L
Tyrosine[b]	Plasma	0.4–1.6	mg/dL	55.19	20–90	µmol/L
Urea nitrogen (BUN)[b]	Serum	8–23	mg/dL	0.0357	2.9–8.2	mmol/L
Uric acid[b]	Serum	4.0–8.5	mg/dL	0.0595	0.24–0.51	mmol/L
Urobilinogen[b]	Urine	0.05–2.5	mg/24 h	1.693	0.1–4.2	µmol/day
Valine[b]	Plasma	1.7–3.7	mg/dL	85.5	145–315	µmol/L
Valproic acid (therapeutic)	Plasma, serum	50–150	µg/mL	6.93	346–1040	µmol/L
Vancomycin (therapeutic)	Plasma, serum	10–20	µg/mL	0.69	6.9–13.8	µmol/L
Vanillylmandelic acid (VMA)[b]	Urine	2.1–7.6	mg/24 h	5.046	11–38	µmol/day
Vasoactive intestinal polypeptide	Plasma	<50	pg/mL	1	<50	ng/L
Verapamil (therapeutic)	Plasma, serum	100–500	ng/mL	2.2	220–1100	nmol/L
Vitamin A (retinol)[b]	Serum	30–80	µg/dL	0.0349	1.05–2.80	µmol/L
Vitamin B$_1$ (thiamine)	Whole blood	2.5–7.5	µg/dL	29.6	74–222	nmol/L
Vitamin B$_2$ (riboflavin)	Plasma, serum	4–24	µg/dL	26.6	106–638	nmol/L
Vitamin B$_5$ (pantothenic acid)	Whole blood	0.2–1.8	µg/mL	4.56	0.9–8.2	µmol/L
Vitamin B$_6$ (pyridoxine)	Plasma	5–30	ng/mL	4.046	20–121	nmol/L
Vitamin B$_{12}$ (cyanocobalamin)[b]	Serum	160–950	pg/mL	0.7378	118–701	pmol/L
Vitamin C (ascorbic acid)	Plasma, serum	0.4–1.5	mg/dL	56.78	23–85	µmol/L
Vitamin D, 1,25-dihydroxyvitamin D	Plasma, serum	16–65	pg/mL	2.6	42–169	pmol/L

	Specimen	Traditional Reference Interval	Traditional Units	Conversion Factor, Multiply →, ← Divide	SI Reference Interval	SI Units
Vitamin D, 25-hydroxyvitamin D	Plasma, serum	14–60	ng/mL	2.496	35–150	nmol/L
Vitamin E (α-tocopherol)[b]	Plasma, serum	0.5–1.8	mg/dL	23.22	12–42	μmol/L
Vitamin K	Plasma, serum	0.13–1.19	ng/mL	2.22	0.29–2.64	nmol/L
von Willebrand factor (ranges vary according to blood type)	Plasma	70–140	%	0.01	0.70–1.40	Fraction of 1.0
Warfarin (therapeutic)	Plasma, serum	1.0–10	μg/mL	3.24	3.2–32.4	μmol/L
White blood cell count[b]	Whole blood	4.5–11.0	$10^3\ \mu L^{-1}$	1	4.5–11.0	$10^9\ L^{-1}$
White blood cell, differential count (see complete blood count)						
Xylose absorption test (25-g dose)[b]	Whole blood	>25 mg/dL	mg/dL	0.06661	>1.7	mmol/L
Zidovudine (therapeutic)	Plasma, serum	0.15–0.27	μg/mL	3.74	0.56–1.01	μmol/L
Zinc	Serum	50–150	μg/dL	0.153	7.7–23.0	μmol/L

The sample type listed under Specimen in this table shows the reference interval for that specimen type. Thus, if the specimen for a test is listed as serum, the reference interval shown is for serum specimens. For many tests listed with serum as the specimen type, plasma is also acceptable, often with a similar reference interval.

The normal ranges listed here are included as a helpful guide and are by no means comprehensive. The listed reference, unless noted, pertains to adults. Laboratory results are method dependent and can have intralaboratory variation. Conversion factors are not affected by age-related differences. This table is compiled from data in the following sources: (1) Tietz NW, ed. *Clinical Guide to Laboratory Tests*. 3rd ed. Philadelphia, PA: WB Saunders Co; 1995; (2) Laposata M. *SI Unit Conversion Guide*. Boston, MA: NEJM Books; 1992; (3) *American Medical Association Manual of Style: A Guide for Authors and Editors*. 9th ed. Chicago, IL: AMA; 1998:486-503. Copyright 1998, American Medical Association; (4) Jacobs DS, DeMott WR, Oxley DK, eds. *Jacobs & DeMott Laboratory Test Handbook with Key Word Index*. 5th ed. Hudson, OH: Lexi-Comp Inc; 2001; (5) Henry JB, ed. *Clinical Diagnosis and Management by Laboratory Methods*. 20th ed. Philadelphia, PA: WB Saunders Co; 2001; (6) Kratz A, et al. Laboratory reference values. *N Engl J Med*. 2006;351:1548-1563; (7) Burtis CA, ed. *Tietz Textbook of Clinical Chemistry and Molecular Diagnostics*. 5th ed. St. Louis, MO: Elsevier; 2012. This version of the table of reference ranges was reviewed and updated by Jessica Franco-Colon, PhD, and Kay Brooks.

[a]The SI unit katal is the amount of enzyme generating 1 mol of product per second. Although provisionally recommended as the SI unit for enzymatic activity, it has not been universally accepted. It is suitable to maintain use of U/L in these circumstances (conversion factor 1.0).

[b]For this analyte, there is sex or age dependence for the reference range. There may be several different normal ranges for different pediatric age groups. Consult your clinical laboratory for the local institution age-specific reference range. Pediatric reference values may also be found in Soldin SJ, Brugnara C, Wong EC, eds.; Hicks JM, editor emeritus. *Pediatric References Intervals*. 5th ed. (formerly *Pediatric Reference Ranges*). Washington, DC: AACC Press; 2005.

Amino Acid	3-Letter Code	1-Letter Code
Alanine	Ala	A
Cysteine	Cys	C
Aspartic acid or aspartate	Asp	D
Glutamic acid or glutamate	Glu	E
Phenylalanine	Phe	F
Glycine	Gly	G
Histidine	His	H
Isoleucine	Ile	I
Lysine	Lys	K
Leucine	Leu	L
Methionine	Met	M
Asparagine	Asn	N
Proline	Pro	P
Glutamine	Gln	Q
Arginine	Arg	R
Serine	Ser	S
Threonine	Thr	T
Valine	Val	V
Tryptophan	Trp	W
Tyrosine	Tyr	Y

Index

Page numbers in bold indicate figures and tables.